The Master Timetable

Junior year January	Choose an advisor and have first meeting.
Mid- March	Plan senior curriculum (including electives).
April	Agreement materials for the NRMP are sent to medical schools.
Mid-June	Student agreement materials for the NRMP for independent applicants are available.
June to July	Prepare preliminary list of programs and meet with your advisor to discuss. Request applications and get application photo taken.
Senior year Mid-July	**Deadline:** NRMP must receive agreement materials from U.S. students, early specialty match materials also due.
July	Request information from residencies on your list. Begin a personal statement and CV.
August	Develop a database, card file, or other method of tracking information and deadlines. Review your personal statement and CV.
September	Request letters of recommendation from faculty. Review your personal statement and CV with your advisor . Begin applications.
Mid- September	The NRMP directory of programs is posted to the Web. Review your list of programs with your advisor.
Mid- October	**Deadline:** Complete submission of applications (deadlines vary, so be careful). Make preliminary inquiries about interviews.
Mid- November	**Deadline:** NRMP must receive agreement materials from independent and sponsored graduate applicants.
November to January	Interview at programs, make notes to yourself.
First week in January	Programs must file final list of quotas and withdrawals. Check for any changes in the programs of interest.
Mid- January	Make and file your Rank Order List.
Mid- February	**Deadline:** Rank Order Lists must be filed by both programs and individuals.
Match day—3	Matched and unmatched information is released to applicants at 12:00 noon eastern standard time (EST).
Match day—2	Filled and unfilled results for individual programs are posted on the Web at 11:30 am EST. Locations of all unfilled positions are released to applicants at 12:00 noon EST. Unmatched applicants may begin contacting unfilled programs at 12:00 noon EST.
Match day	Match results are given out at 12:00 noon EST. Match results are posted on the NRMP Web site at 1:00 p.m. EST.
March to Mid-April	Letters of appointment or agreement are sent to the student and must be returned.

From Medical School to Residency

Springer
New York
Berlin
Heidelberg
Barcelona
Hong Kong
London
Milan
Paris
Singapore
Tokyo

Roger P. Smith, M.D.

Professor and Program Director
Director of Ambulatory Care
Department of Obstetrics and Gynecology
University of Missouri at Kansas City—Truman Medical Center
Kansas City, Missouri, USA

From Medical School to Residency

How to Compete Successfully in the Residency Match Program

With 57 Illustrations

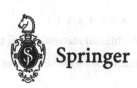
Springer

Roger P. Smith, M.D.
Professor and Program Director
Director of Ambulatory Care
Department of Obstetrics and Gynecology
University of Missouri at Kansas City—Truman Medical Center
2301 Holmes Street
Kansas City, MO 64108
USA

Library of Congress Cataloging-in-Publication Data
Smith, Roger P. (Roger Perry), 1949–
    From medical school to residency : how to compete successfully in the residency match
program / Roger P. Smith.
        p.   cm. —
    Includes bibliographical references and index.
    ISBN 0-387-95003-6 (softcover : alk. paper)
    1. Medical education.   2. Medicine—Study and teaching (Residency).   I. Title: How to
compete successfully in the residency match program.   II. Title.
    [DNLM: 1.   Education, Medical, Graduate—United States.   2.   Internship and
Residency—United States. W20 S658f 2000]
    R737.S5767   2000
    610°.71°55—dc21   00-024951

Printed on acid-free paper.

Production managed by MaryAnn Brickner; manufacturing supervised by Jerome Basma.
Photocomposed copy prepared from the author's Microsoft Word files.
Printed and bound by Hamilton Printing Co., Rensselaer, NY.
Printed in the United States of America.

9 8 7 6 5 4 3 2 1

Additional material to this book can be downloaded from http://extras.springer.com.

ISBN 0-387-95003-6 Springer-Verlag New York Berlin Heidelberg   SPIN 10755982

Preface

Medical graduates seeking training in the United States get their residency assignment through a matching process managed by the National Residency Matching Program (NRMP). The process is intimidating for most; traumatic for some. However, there are tips that can make the task easier and increase the likelihood of success. Many of these tips are known to those of us who advise students or are involved in the resident selection process, but this only helps if students have access to a good advisor, and not everyone does. This text is designed to fill that need for the student without access and to supplement the advice received for those who do.

No text can provide final answers to questions that are inherently subjective—only you, the student, can pose and answer those questions. The intent of this text is to help you frame those questions, develop strategies to assess them, and, finally, feel comfortable with your final decision. This book provides a glimpse into what residencies look for, how to choose the right program for yourself, and the sequence of tasks you must accomplish to navigate the process. It is easy to believe that everyone else is better, faster, bigger, and after exactly the spot you want. This book gives you the tools you need to ensure that you can be anybody's match.

Contents

Chapter 1
Graduate Medical Education
and "The Match"

Anybody's Match

It won't be that long before you join the over 15,000 medical students who are awarded the M.D. degree each year at one of 125 medical schools. Unfortunately, this does not qualify you to practice medicine; you still have a ways to go. Before you can hang out your shingle or put you name on the door, you have to complete an additional three to seven years of residency training (one to three years just to be licensed in most states). In a manner somewhat akin to the process you went through getting in to college and medical school, you now face choosing where this training will take place and in what field of practice. Since 1952, this process has been simplified somewhat by the institution of a national system designed to match candidates and programs. A similar program is in place for graduates of schools of osteopathic medicine as well. This system also provides for a uniform decision date; further reducing the stress of the process. The system is designed to level the playing field, allowing students to obtain the most desirable position available to them. (Over 80% get their first, second, or third choice.) Almost all graduate medical trainees in the United States go through the matching process to get their residency assignment. There are some individual specialties and special circumstances that have their own version of the matching process, and these will be discussed in Chapter 15.

This is not to say that the system is either simple or stress-free. It is not. The process is intimidating for most, traumatic for some. There are, however, some tips and guidelines that can be provided to make the task easier and that will increase your chances of success. Many of these are well known to those who advise students or who are involved in the resident selection process, but they are only available to students if they have access to a good mentor. This text should fill that need for students without access and supplement the advice received by those who have an advisor.

Despite the National Resident Matching Program (NRMP, the match), there are many decisions still to be made, forms to be filed, interviews to be arranged and undergone, and lastly, the ranking of your choices and the match itself. How can you make this process smoother, less intimidating, and successful in getting you to your ideal residency? This book can provide you with a road map, battle plan, time line, and helpful hints to ease the way. No text can provide final answers to questions that are inherently subjective—only you can pose and answer those questions. The intent of this text is to help you frame those questions, develop strategies to assess them, and ultimately feel comfortable with your final decision.

In the chapters that follow, we will explore the graduate medical education system and the application process. We will look at ways to decide on your field of study, and the type of residency you might want, and to assess your chances of getting an appointment to the program of your choice. We will move through the various steps that you will have to traverse on your journey to that ideal position, providing hint, tricks, and the benefit of experience along the way. While we will explore the options available if you do not match, the odds are vastly in your favor that you will not need them. Let us begin by looking at the process of postgraduate medical education.

Postgraduate Education

There is no single licensure to practice medicine throughout the United States; however, there are broad standards that the individual states adhere to in granting medical licensure. To provide patient care in the United States, a physician must complete several years of postgraduate study in an approved graduate medical education program. Programs are accredited by the Accreditation Council for Graduate Medical Education (ACGME) and must meet standards set by the certifying boards within each medical specialty. These boards specify the formal training required, set the standards for certification, administer the testing that determines that these standards have been met, and oversee the work of the residency review committees (RRCs) for their specialty. The duration of postgraduate medical education determined by the individual specialty boards, but ranges from three to seven years (Figure 1-1).

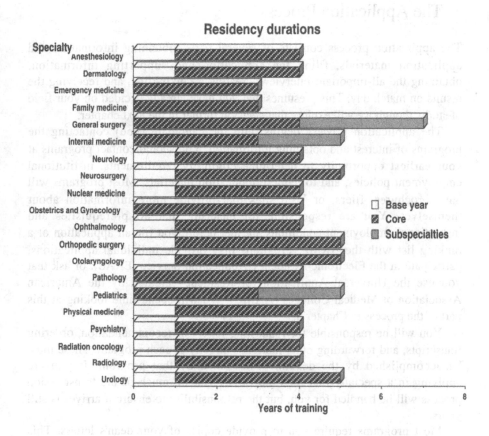

Figure 1-1 Many specialties combine the base year into the core program but may still allow a candidate to enter after a preliminary medicine or transitional year. The base year for surgical specialties consists of general surgery. If you are considering a program that requires a preliminary year, you often have to apply for the advanced training at the same time.

There are approximately 80,000 physicians in residency or fellowship training programs at any time. There are currently 3,879 residency programs at over 700 teaching hospitals offering over 24,200 individual positions. These programs range from small to large and can be found everywhere from modest-sized communities to large university centers. There is no best residency just as there is no best field of medical practice, best automobile, or best Italian restaurant. "Best" is subjective. Fortunately, for the majority of graduates from United States and Canadian medical schools, there are generally enough options to go around.

The Application Process

The application process consists of several parts: obtaining information and application materials, filing the application and supporting information, obtaining the all-important interview, creating a ranking list, and receiving the results on match day. This presumes that you have already decided on your field of study, though we will explore that decision further in the next chapter.

The application process begins with the candidate (you) contacting the programs of interest and obtaining information. You should contact programs at your earliest opportunity to determine eligibility requirements, institutional employment policies, and to request application materials. Most programs will have brochures, fliers, or Web sites that provide more information about themselves. You are responsible for ensuring that all prerequisites and institutional employment conditions are met before you file an application or a ranking list with the NRMP. Programs may provide individual applications, participate in the Electronic Residency Application Service (ERAS), or ask that you use the Universal Application for Residency created by the American Association of Medical Colleges (AAMC). We will spend time looking at this part of the process in Chapter 8.

You will be responsible for requesting letters of recommendation, ordering transcripts, and forwarding other materials directly to each program. These must be accomplished by the deadline established by that program. If you are applying in a specialty that uses the ERAS system, much of the transmission process will be handled for you, but the responsibility to ensure it arrives is still yours.

Most programs require you to provide copies of your dean's letters. This letter is the standard recommendation prepared by U.S. medical schools on behalf of their graduating seniors. In place of the dean's letters, graduates from other medical schools must provide recommendations from individuals capable of evaluating their potential as physicians. This will most often be senior faculty from their medical school. Even if you have a dean's letters, you will probably need letters of recommendation and evaluation from two to three additional faculty. In Chapter 11, we will look at this aspect of the process in detail.

As the applications come in, program directors review the candidates' credentials and, if interested, will extend invitations for interviews. During the months of October though January, candidates and programs meet each other in this process and determine their list of preferences, known as their "rank order list." Once these lists are filed with the NRMP, the computers match everyone up. Through this process, each candidate receives an appointment to the residency with the highest position possible on his or her list.

Types of Residencies

Residencies take several forms. There are programs that are based in community hospitals, programs that are affiliated with a university or medical center, and those that are located in and run by a university. There are programs with just a few trainees and others with veritable armies of housestaff. There are programs that stress preparation for advanced subspecialty training (fellowships) and those that specialize in producing practicing physicians. This palette of choices ensures that there is at least one option that will meet your needs.

To add to this list of variations, the NRMP recognizes three types of positions: Preliminary, Categorical, and Specialty (Table 1-1). The NRMP designations are the formal ones, while the other characterizations are more subjective. For the most part, the decision to apply to a preliminary or categorical program will be driven by your choice of medical specialty and the certainty of your plans.

Many students (and advisors) make a great distinction between community-based programs and those offered by university centers. This distinction is more imagined and stylistic than real. While we will look at this issue in detail in Chapters 2 and 4, be assured that the standards set by the ACGME, with oversight carried out by the individual specialty boards, ensures that the training in each residency meets the same standards. That is to say, styles differ, but the content is the same (within the same specialty).

Table 1-1 Types of Positions Offered Through the National Residency Match Program

- Preliminary positions provide one or two years of prerequisite training for entry into an advanced positions in specialty programs that require one or more years of broad clinical training. Internal medicine, surgery, and transitional programs commonly offer preliminary positions.
- Categorical positions are in programs that expect applicants who enter in their first postgraduate year to continue until they have completed all of the training required for specialty certification.
- Specialty positions (beginning in 2000) are in positions that begin after completion of one or more years of preliminary training. Starting in 1999, applicants without prior graduate medical education have had the option to apply for these positions while also applying for preliminary positions.

Fields of Study

There are twenty-five areas of specialization that offer board certification (Table 1-2). In some cases, these represent segments of a larger field (such as branches of surgery such as orthopedics, vascular surgery, or urology). In other cases, such as pathology, obstetrics and gynecology, or family medicine, the programs are self-contained entities that do not require or accept preliminary or transitional experience as credit toward certification. Within many of these fields there are subspecialization options available either as specific residency programs or as postgraduate fellowships.

Table 1-2 Medical Specialty Boards

Allergy and immunology	Orthopedic surgery
Anesthesiology	Otolaryngology
Colon and rectal surgery	Pathology
Dermatology	Pediatrics
Emergency medicine	Physical medicine
Family medicine	Plastic surgery
General surgery	Preventive medicine
Internal medicine	Psychiatry and neurology
Medical genetics	Radiology
Neurologic surgery	Surgery
Nuclear medicine	Thoracic surgery
Obstetrics and gynecology	Urology
Ophthalmology	

Each field of medical study has its own style. Each residency entails its own forms of pleasure and stress. No field of study is easier or harder than any other, so only you can decide your best fit. In the next chapter, we will explore this aspect of your choices.

The Match

At one time, finding a residency was like entering a college or medical school—with staggered acceptances, different deadlines, and lists of those awaiting admission. As noted above, since 1952 the process has been made easier by the institution of the NRMP match. Today almost everyone looking for a residency goes through the matching process. The 1999 main match placed 20,170 applicants for postgraduate medical training positions into 3,775 residency programs at 701 teaching hospitals throughout the United States. (This represents over 98% of programs and 97% of students.) The 2000 match is expected to involve over 24,200 positions of various types. Applicants and residency programs evaluate and rank one another, and then a computerized process pairs applicants with programs based on the ranked preferences. The NRMP also conducts matches for fellowship positions, through its Specialties Matching Services. These positions involve further training beyond completion of the initial residency program and lead to certification in a subspecialty (e.g., cardiology). These fellowship matches are made throughout the year and go through a separate process.

The match process is designed to maximize the process for all involved. Residency programs want the best and the brightest to represent them as graduates and challenge them as trainees. Medical schools want to see their graduates get the best positions possible for the prestige and status they bring. It also helps to assure incoming medical students of their future ability to pursue postgraduate training. Most importantly, it maximizes the ability of the student to be placed in the most desirable program possible, enhancing satisfaction, self-esteem, and future prosperity.

Despite the goals of the match, approximately 8% of United States and Canadian graduates and up to 60% of foreign graduates fail to match to a position, while 15% of positions go unfilled. This occurs for a variety of reasons: Some candidates apply to or rank too few programs. They rank programs to which they are not well suited. They fail to use the system in their favor, or they fail to make a strong case for their candidacy. Most of these failings are easily avoided.

This, then, is what it is all about—matching up your strengths and weaknesses, your likes and desires, with the best possible training position in the field of medicine you have chosen. While the decisions you will make are not irrevocable or immutable, they are sufficiently important to warrant your full attention. With some common sense, helpful hints, and simple strategies, you, too, can be anybody's match.

Chapter 2
Choosing Residencies

The one decision that is pivotal to finding a residency is, What field of medicine do you want to pursue? This affects everything from the duration of training to its location. If your goal is to be a pediatric cardiologist, you are in for a long haul in a major medical center. If you want to be a family medicine specialist, your have a shorter training program and more options for geographic location and program size. How do you go about choosing? Or, if you have already decided what you want to be when you grow up, how do you decide if your choice is really the best for you? Most of the time, this is a decision of the heart, not the head. There are, however, things you can do to remove some of the heartburn.

Styles and Contents

Think about the qualities of the department or specialty you are considering. There are specialties that prize cognitive and contemplative processes, others demand decisiveness and assertion. Some allow professional and personal lives that are ordered and controlled; others are unpredictable and chaotic. You have probably noticed these differences, and these may have been the factors that drew you to a career in your chosen field. (To hear the stereotypes, just listen to the jokes told in the surgeons' lounge or at a medicine conference.)

The earlier in your clinical years you make a choice about career, the less pressure there is, but there is a greater chance that you will find something else that attracts you further along in the process. There is no ideal time to choose, no deadline to meet. Indeed, a few will not have chosen by the time they graduate. These students can hedge their options by taking a transitional or preliminary year while they consider the problem. The decision comes earlier and easier to some than to others. You can use senior-year electives to explore alternatives or reinforce a decision, but only if these are taken at the beginning of the senior year. If you have not been able to settle on a field by the fall of your senior year, a transitional option, research, or an advanced degree (M.P.H.) is your safest choice.

Even if your selection seems preordained, a bit of reappraisal is still in order. Are the role models you have encountered representative of the field in general? This may be difficult for students to decide on their own: Ask around. Ask others in the field if your idols have the respect of their peers? Are they active on the regional or national level? Do they sit on committees in their department, school, or state? Is this the norm for the specialty, or are the people you have encountered over- or underachievers?

Are the activities you observe in the hospital setting representative of the professional activities practiced in your field? Do you have a sense of the professional rewards and frustrations unique to your specialty? If you are unsure, ask. Ask residents why they chose the way they did. Are they still happy with that decision? Ask faculty and local practitioners the same thing.

Once you decide what qualities someone in your field has, how do you measure up? Here, brutal honesty is the gentlest course. Do you really have that same demeanor, make decisions in the same way, like working the same hours? Ask your friends to tell you if they can see you in the role. Your friends will let you know. (As in other areas, laughter may be the best medicine—it may cure you of an ill-advised decision.) If they don't think you fit the mold, you may want to recognize the uphill nature of the task ahead and reevaluate. Don't give up on a dream; just be prepared to dig in. The bottom line is that it is your decision to make.

When you look at the residents and faculty of the department you have selected, do they seem like "your kind of people?" Are they similar to the friends you have chosen? (The style of those you choose as friends reflects your characteristics.) Would you enjoy working with these people? They will be asking themselves the same question about you during the process. Remember that the match is a two-way process. You select them just as much or more than they select you.

If you have a spouse or significant other, (especially one that will be following you in your further training) include them in this decision. Their career and life plans will have an impact on your choices. If your partner also in medicine, how will your professional paths interact? Look at everything, from at-home consultations to office hours, call schedules to philosophy and practice style. Will your spouse or significant other understand the joys you derive from your profession and will you value theirs?

After Residency

Another factor you will want to consider when you decide on possible training programs is your plan for after the residency. Do you plan a career of practice, academics, research, or administration? If you want to be a captain of the health care industry, choosing a residency in an institution that also offers advanced business degrees is wise. If you plan to follow your residency with fellowship training, look for a residency that either offers a fellowship in your field or has a good record of accomplishment for fellowship placement.

All residencies should prepare you for certification in your field. There is, however, some variation in the degree of success various programs enjoy. The program director in each program receives annual reports from their certifying board on how their graduates do each year. These reports are confidential and even the program director does not know the identity of the candidates, just how they did. The program directors or their staff can give you an idea of how their candidates did, though this is often the nebulous "they all do fine." If pressed, they should be able to give a more specific answer. (This is a good question to ask during your interview.)

Are you considering a subspecialty or specialized career outside of the mainstream of fields represented in medical schools? These fascinating branches of medicine should not be overlooked. If you are considering these fields, you will need to consider preliminary training that prepares you for the advanced programs and experience needed for certification. (A list of some of these options, with their certifying boards, is given in Table 2-1.)

Table 2-1 Subspecialty Certification or Special Qualifications

Specialty	Certifying board
Addiction psychiatry	Psychiatry and Neurology
Adolescent medicine	Internal Medicine
	Pediatrics
Aerospace medicine	Preventive Medicine
Anatomic and clinical pathology	Pathology
Anatomic pathology	Pathology
Blood bank	Pathology
Transfusion medicine	
Cardiovascular disease	Internal Medicine
Chemical pathology	Pathology
Child and adolescent psychiatry	Psychiatry and Neurology
Clinical biochemical genetics	Medical Genetics
Clinical cardiac electrophysiology	Internal Medicine
Clinical cytogenetics	Medical Genetics
Clinical genetics	Medical Genetics
Clinical and laboratory dermatologic immunology	Dermatology
Clinical and laboratory immunology	Allergy and Immunology
	Internal Medicine
	Pediatrics
Clinical molecular genetics	Medical Genetics
Clinical neurophysiology	Psychiatry and Neurology
Clinical pathology	Pathology

Colon and rectal surgery	Colon and Rectal Surgery
Critical care medicine	Anesthesiology Internal Medicine
Cytopathology	Pathology
Dermatopathology	Dermatology Pathology
Diagnostic radiology	Radiology
Endocrinology, diabetes, and metabolic disease	Internal Medicine
Forensic pathology	Pathology
Forensic psychiatry	Psychiatry and Neurology
Gastroenterology	Internal Medicine
General vascular surgery	Surgery
Geriatric medicine	Family Practice Internal Medicine
Geriatric psychiatry	Psychiatry and Neurology
Gynecologic oncology	Obstetrics and Gynecology
Hand surgery	Orthopedic surgery Plastic Surgery
Hematology	Internal Medicine Pathology
Immunopathology	Pathology
Infectious diseases	Internal Medicine
Maternal and fetal medicine	Obstetrics and Gynecology
Medical genetics	Medical Genetics
Medical microbiology	Pathology
Medical oncology	Internal Medicine
Medical toxicology	Emergency Medicine Pediatrics Preventive Medicine
Neonatal-perinatal medicine	Pediatrics
Nephrology	Internal Medicine
Neurology with special qualifications in child neurology	Psychiatry and Neurology
Neurology	Psychiatry and Neurology
Neuropathology	Pathology
Neuroradiology	Radiology
Occupational medicine	Preventive Medicine
Otology neurotology	Otolaryngology
Pain management	Anesthesiology
Pediatric cardiology	Pediatrics
Pediatric critical care medicine	Pediatrics
Pediatric emergency medicine	Emergency Medicine Pediatrics

Pediatric endocrinology	Pediatrics
Pediatric gastroenterology	Pediatrics
Pediatric hematology-oncology	Pediatrics
Pediatric infectious diseases	Pediatrics
Pediatric nephrology	Pediatrics
Pediatric otology	Otolaryngology
Pediatric pathology	Pathology
Pediatric pulmonology	Pediatrics
Pediatric radiology	Pediatrics
	Radiology
Pediatric surgery	Surgery
Psychiatry	Psychiatry and Neurology
Public health and general preventive medicine	Preventive Medicine
Pulmonary disease	Internal Medicine
Radiation oncology	Radiology
Radiological physics	Radiology
Reproductive medicine	Obstetrics and Gynecology
Rheumatology	Internal Medicine
Spinal cord injury medicine	Physical Medicine and
	Rehabilitation
Sports medicine	Emergency Medicine
	Family Practice
	Internal Medicine
	Pediatrics
Surgery of the hand	Surgery
Surgical critical care	Surgery
Underseas medicine	Preventive Medicine
Urogynecology and pelvic floor surgery	Obstetrics and Gynecology
Vascular interventional radiology	Radiology

While geographic and job portability are greater than they once were, you should consider where you might want to locate after your residency is through. During your residency, you may begin putting down family and professional roots that make relocation outside the region more difficult. Marriage, children, your parents, in-laws, and others may define the region where you train or where you stay after the residency ends. While you are in training, you will develop relationships with other physicians in your field. These will form the core of your professional support and referral networks. You will learn the character of local and regional practices, making it easier to decide those you admire and those you would want to avoid. These factors, too, tend to tie you to an area, so look at the long-term as well as the short-tern when thinking of residency options.

Location, Location

No area is better or worse for residency training, establishing a practice, or living. Most of the time, geographic decisions will revolve around personal preference and point of view (Figure 2-1). You may prefer to stay near where you grew up, or explore new vistas. You may be influenced by past visits, childhood vacations, hobbies, weather patterns, or sports preferences. (If you like water sports, Albuquerque is not a good choice.) I even know of a young woman who enjoyed NASCAR racing, working as a volunteer on pit crews. One of her criteria for a residency was that it had to be within an hour's drive of a NASCAR race course. That is as good a way to pick residencies as any other. Consider the options carefully because you will be spending several years in this location and you will need to have a life outside of the hospital (and so will any family you have).

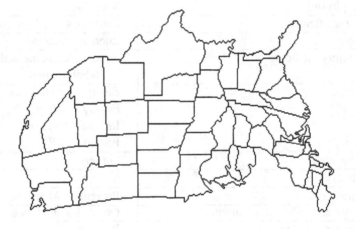

Figure 2-1 A Canadian medical student's view of United States residencies.

If you are thinking of a residency outside the region of your medical or undergraduate schools, and you have not had any experience living in that area, consider a vacation or clinical rotation before you make a final choice. You may have always heard of the locale's hospitality or warmth, but if you arrive to find you are treated as a Yankee, hick, or city slicker you may be less than happy with your choice. Check on the Internet for information about travel or tourism in the area that you are considering. The local Chamber of Commerce can often give you a feel for the area. One trick you can use to learn about a city is to look at a local phone book, either in your library or while you visit for an interview. Look up goods or services that you might use. Do they have a bowling alley? An art gallery? How many movie theaters are there? Are the only car dealers Lexus dealers? Where can you get pet food for your pet iguana? You get the idea.

Your field of medicine and style of practice may affect the location options available to you when you finish your training and, by extension, where you may want to look for a residency. For example, assume that you want to specialize in geriatrics. While the Great Plains have their share of retirees, the ability to build a thriving practice is not as great as it would be in Sun City. In your field, is a geographic area over- or underserved? If your plan to practice, do you want a solo practice, to be part of a group, or to be employed by a health maintenance organization? Even these choices can affect locale to some extent.

A consideration for many students is the employment opportunities available for a spouse or significant other. The more general your partner's vocation or skills, the less this may be a factor. For both logistic and interpersonal reasons, address this early in your contemplation. Don't forget when you go out on the interview trail to take your partner along, even if an interview for him or her is not available or appropriate. (The special circumstances of the two-physician medical family and the "couples match" are addressed in Chapter 15.)

Competitiveness

This aspect of choosing a field of study or picking a residency is more subjective and more uncomfortable because it requires brutal self-assessment. Competitiveness refers not to your willingness to join the intramural tug-of-war team, but to the selection process of the match. A competitive residency program is one that is highly respected and sought after, resulting in many qualified applicants for a few positions. This means that the program can select whom it wants. (The match is driven by the candidate's rank order list, but when there are a large number of qualified candidates who all rank a program highly, the program is more likely to get its first choices.) In a similar way, a competitive candidate is one who is highly qualified, motivated, personable, and desirable. The essence of the match is making sure that both parties feel that the other was the most desirable option.

You can gauge the competitiveness of a residency program is several ways: Did the program fill all of its available slots in the last match? (Table 2-2) In very popular fields, this may not discriminate well because all of the slots may fill in even the less desirable programs. You must also realize that a field with a 97% match rate may still result in 15% to 20% of candidates not matching because of poor planning or unrealistic expectations.

Table 2-2 Number of Unmatched Slots in 1999

Anesthesiology	75	Orthopedic surgery	2
Dermatology	0	Otolaryngology	4
Emergency medicine	30	Pathology	63
Family medicine	561	Pediatrics (all)[*]	27
General surgery (all)[*]	466	Physical medicine	9
Internal medicine (all)[*]	470	Psychiatry	51
Neurology	6	Radiation oncology	2
Neurosurgery	1	Radiology	9
Obstetrics and gynecology	78	Transitional	55
Ophthalmology	1	Urology	7

*Includes preliminary (postgraduate year 1 only) and first-year categorical positions.

If your school has placed residents in a program in the past, were they only the best of the class? Has your school been successful in getting someone in at all? How do your advisors or faculty members in that field perceive the program? You can ask a program how many applications it received in the last cycle, but remember that even the poorest program will often interview ten to twenty applicants for each position and have applications from many more. Keep in mind that the program's reputation, good or bad, may not be deserved.

The most difficult, and often painful, part of the competitiveness question is your competitiveness as a candidate. This is somewhat independent of your field of interest. Some of the components of competitiveness you already know: How have your medical school grades been so far? Have you gotten good comments on your clinical rotations? How have you done on the United States Medical Licensure (USMLE, "the boards") examinations? Are there any problems that will have to be explained or highlights to be showcased? Your best source of guidance in this area will be your advisor. He or she will be able to give an objective assessment of your chances in the field you are considering. Under some circumstances, he or she may even suggest a reconsideration of your goals or expectations (up or down). Your advisor will be able to suggest areas that can be strengthen or highlighted. This role is so important that we will devote an entire chapter to the advising process (Chapter 5).

Does Size Really Matter?

Whether its residencies or fries, sometimes bigger isn't necessarily better. Like location, there is no right answer as to how big a residency program should be. Small programs offer an intimacy that can be lost in larger numbers. You are likely to get to know your faculty and attending physicians well, learning in an almost apprenticeship-like environment. You will generally have fewer faculty members to draw experience from, and smaller programs often have a lighter patient load. Fewer patients may mean a more relaxed pace, but not always, and will limit the number of exotic cases you are likely to encounter. This is more of a problem in subspecialties than in general fields. Smaller programs are often found in smaller health centers that may lack the bells and whistles of the high-tech corporate research centers.

Residencies with large numbers of residents have more hands to help with the work, but have more work to do. Call schedules may be slightly lighter, but more intense. You will have more faculty members to draw on, but potentially be more isolated from them. Large programs are most often located in major referral centers, thus receiving more complicated and unusual cases. This benefits the subspecialists but does not detract from the experience of more general pursuits. While small programs may be found in metropolitan areas, large residencies are usually restricted to referral centers located in urban settings.

Your decisions about location may already provide some constraints on residency size. If you have decided on a rural lifestyle, chances are that you will be looking at smaller programs than if you like the bright lights of the big city. Some fields of study are only offered in a limited number of locations, though there is generally a range of program sizes from which to choose.

The Myth of "The" Residency

Every field has its Mayo Clinics, M. D. Andersons, Kaiser Permanentes, and others whose names are synonymous with special care, innovative research, distinguished programs and the like. In each field, some programs carry reputations that make them the pinnacle to which all others strive - "the" place to train at. Even physicians in other fields can often name these institutions of renown. However, does this mean that this sort of institution is where you should train? The answer is easy: don't worry about it. There are lots of good places in each and every field of medicine; there is no best.

To be a certified residency in any field of medicine, a training program must meet certain standardized criteria laid out by that specialty's certifying board. Each board sets standards for the academic content and experience opportunities required for training in their field. Residency review committees (RRCs) that serve under the direction of these boards evaluate programs based on these criteria. It is the task of the RRC to periodically assess each program and certify that the criteria are met or exceeded. Consequently, any certified program in a given field of medicine, by definition, must provide the same minimum level of experience as any other. There are styles and flourishes to be sure, but the minimum training necessary to become certified must be present. While there may be some level of prestige associated with being a graduate of "Old Pooh-

Pooh U.", we all know that only goes so far. That isn't to say that if you want to go on to a fellowship or an academic appointment after residency the name of your alma matter won't help - it will, but only to get you the interview. After that, it is up to you.

The message is, Choose your residency based on other factors first and name or reputation second. Just because a program has a big name, don't rank it above others you like better. Just because a program has a big name, don't shy away from it either. Name is only one factor, not "the" factor.

How Many?

The minimum number of programs you should plan on applying to will be dependent on a number of factors. You will need to consider the competitiveness of the field you are entering, your desirability as a candidate, and any special circumstances that statistically reduce your chance of success (couples match, independent candidate, foreign graduate). One crude method of estimating a working minimum number of programs is the simple formula:

Minimum number of programs = 5 + 5•(SF) + 5•(CR) + 5•(CM) + 10•(FG)

SF = Specialty Factor (1 - easy, 2 - average, 3 - highly competitive)

CR = Class Rank (1 - first third, 2 - second third, 3 - last third)

CM = Couples Match (1 - yes, 0 - no)

FG = Foreign Graduate (1 - yes, 0 - no)

You can see by this method that a gifted single U.S. student who is seeking a position in a less competitive field would only need to apply to a minimum of fifteen or so programs. An average student who wants a moderately competitive field would need to apply to more than twenty-five residencies. This is a starting number and provides a starting place for you and your advisor to refine further. Factors that would reduce your flexibility or reduce your desirability as a candidate should increase this number further. Examples might include the need to be located in a specific area of the country or uncertain career plans.

The mixture of programs to put on your list will also be driven, in part, by your desirability as a candidate (Table 2-3). All students should spread their applications among programs of varied desirability and competitiveness. The proportion you use should be determined in consultation with your advisor.

Table 2-3 Guidelines for Program Mixtures (Proportion of Total)

	Program Competitiveness		
Class standing	**High**	**Moderate**	**Low**
Top third	2/5	2/5	1/5
Middle third	1/5	3/5	1/5
Lower third	-	2/5	3/5*

* Should also include some transitional or preliminary options from your plan B

Plan B

The majority of students involved in the match process will obtain a position in their chosen field. No matter how good your qualifications, character, and résumé, there is a chance that you may not be successful in the match. This can happen because you have ranked too few programs, your expectations were unrealistic, or you did not do a good job of matching to the styles of the programs you listed. This is not a value judgment and it does not reflect on your worth or ability to be a physician; it is just a mismatch.

If really good candidates occasionally end up unmatched, what about the rest of us? This is where plan B comes in. Before you complete your assessment of possible residencies, think about what you would do if you don't match. Do you want to be part of the scramble for any unfilled positions, or would you want to do a transitional year? This is your plan B.

Some specialties have few or no unmatched positions, while others have more positions than students. This can even change over time (Figure 2-2). Some fields of medicine encourage a preliminary or transitional year; others will not extend credit for these studies. Which option is best for you? There is no absolute answer since it will depend on your preferred field, your sense of your competitiveness, and your risk tolerance. If you just have to be a member of a given specialty, at any cost, roll the dice and take your chances in the scramble in the unlikely event your are unmatched. If you are less certain of your field of choice, less competitive, or like the security of a safety net, plan to interview and rank one or more transitional programs as a backup.

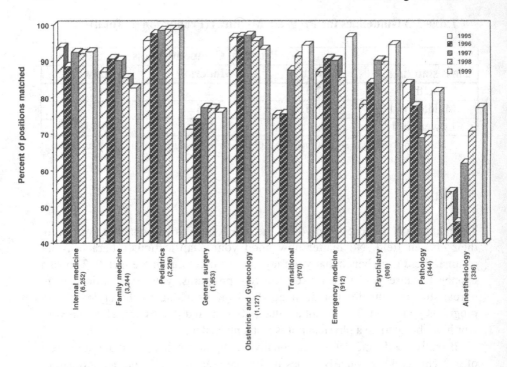

Figure 2-2 The percentage of first year positions filled through the match for the ten most popular specialties. The number shown in parentheses is the number of positions offered in 1999.

An alternative to the transitional year is to consider a related or similar field. For example, suppose you are considering going into obstetrics and gynecology. As a backup, you might consider family medicine because those practitioners do many of the same things (with the exception of surgical therapy). If you want to be a cardiovascular surgeon, could you be happy as a cardiologist? Could you benefit from extra experience in internal medicine or family medicine? Would a year or two of research interest you? Have you ever considered going for an M.P.H. or Ph.D.? Sometimes there is a "backdoor" route. This occurs when more than one discipline offers the same content, such as sports medicine, immunology, or adolescent medicine. Review the list of programs and slots offered and look for these often-overlooked options (Table 2-4).

If your plan B will involve one or more backup programs, you will need to apply and interview at these in the same way that you do for your primary choice. While honesty is always best, telling these programs that you are somewhat undecided is better than telling them they are last on your list.

Table 2-4

Program	Programs participating	Positions offered
Anesthesiology	188	1,083
Dermatology	100	252
Emergency Medicine	120	1,122
Family Practice	518	3,382
Family Practice–Psychiatry	10	17
Internal Medicine–Categorical	375	5,296
Internal Medicine–Emergency Medicine	8	19
Internal Medicine–Family Practice	2	8
Internal Medicine–Neurology	4	6
Internal Medicine–Pediatrics	104	454
Internal Medicine–Physical Medicine and Rehabilitation	5	8
Internal Medicine–Preliminary	259	1,523
Internal Medicine–Primary	91	676
Internal Medicine–Psychiatry	23	49
Neurological Surgery	24	34
Neurology	21	54
Nuclear Medicine	5	7
Obstetrics-Gynecology	251	1136
Ophthalmology	4	9
Orthopedic Surgery	154	560
Otolaryngology	20	44
Pathology	144	450
Pediatrics	184	2,179
Pediatrics–Emergency Medicine	2	4
Pediatrics–Physical Medicine and Rehabilitation	6	6
Pediatrics–Primary	19	149
Pediatrics/Psychiatry/Child Psychiatry	10	20
Physical Medicine and Rehabilitation	93	324
Plastic Surgery	27	51
Preventive Medicine/Public Health	8	16
Psychiatry	199	1,079
Psychiatry–Child Psychiatry	5	10
Psychiatry–Neurology	4	5
Radiation–Oncology	60	96
Radiology–Diagnostic	213	887
Surgery–Categorical	245	1,046
Surgery–Plastic Surgery	15	24
Surgery–Preliminary	201	1005
Transitional	128	1053
Urology	30	62
Total	3,879	24,205

Chapter 3
Choosing Residents; Choosing You

To maximize your chances of matching to *the* residency, you must understand what residencies are looking for and package yourself accordingly. No, this is not to suggest that you should be someone you are not. Fibbing by either party will result in disappointment on both sides. It is about packaging, advertising, and marketing your strengths. It is about finding a *match* between you and the residency. To do this requires some sense of what they are seeking and how they go about the process. This glimpse can help crystallize an image of what you should be seeking from them as well.

Who Are They Looking For?

To answer this question, put yourself in their shoes: Think about the things that make a good resident in general, and then consider the things that would make for a good resident in your chosen field or institution. Once you have a feel for who they need or want, you can look at your own style, experiences, strengths, and weaknesses to decide on the best fit.

It does not require much imagination to envision what makes a good resident. The most successful residents are those who are personable, eager, and self-motivated. They are fun to interact with, to teach, and to learn from. Good people skills and a sense of purpose keep them focused but in perspective. People who know how to work hard but also how to decompress, relax, and keep stress at bay will be happier and most successful in the fast-paced environment that is the majority of residencies.

Selection committees look for someone who would be enjoyable to work with. Not the life-of-the-party type, but rather someone they can get along with, someone it would be fun and challenging to have as a colleague, someone who is an interested learner. What type of people do you like to work with? People who are happy with their field of study, work environment, and life's lot are a pleasure to have around; others are not. Now you get the idea.

As we discussed in the preceding chapter, each specialty in medicine has its style, function, pace, and some might say charm. Within each specialty, however, there is still wide variation in the character of individual educational programs: some are stiff and regimented, some warm and fuzzy. Programs tend to perpetuate these individual styles over time, and will tend to look for candidates that match their characteristics.

What Do They Like?

Most residency programs look for candidates with evidence of integrity, industry, and diversity. Selection committees like students who have broadened their experience with outside activities or leadership positions. Balance is the key. All work and no play can be bad, but all play and no work can be fatal to your chances of selection in the most selective programs. Committees look at the big picture; a last-minute push to get on the school paper, start a homeless shelter, and cure AIDS will probably be seen for what it is—a nice try, too late. For this reason, it is appropriate to draw on significant outside activities you have been involved with from the start of college onward. These should be listed in the appropriate places on you application and curriculum vitae.

Employment or research experience is often touted as important to get you noticed; in general, these are overrated. Yes, the maturity gained in the work force and the intellectual challenges provided by working in a research environment are positive life experiences. Yes, they do suggest reliability. Yes, they do support an image of industry and initiative. No, the committee does not believe that most candidates have been captains of industry or directed the research in which they participated. As educators, we are looking for potential, not necessarily accomplishments. We know that most of the time these were part-time, entry-level experiences. Positive, but not a reason you have to go out and get a job for the summer. A directed summer educational experience (Europe with a purpose) will do just as nicely.

What about gender, racial, and regional bias? Because of the way the computerized matching process works, it is almost impossible to stack the deck successfully in favor of more men, fewer whites, or more Yankees. Yes, programs do like diversity of all kinds. No program wants to become populated only by its own medical students. Similarly, to have no students stay on in your residency is equally bad. Therefore, while balance in all of its many forms is desirable, there really isn't much the selection committee can do to change it short of closing its doors to one group or another. With the matching system, you have as good a chance as anyone else—no favorites, no penalties.

Do the resident selection committees seek out "known commodities"? Does it help to spend time in the department or do an elective in it? While we will devote much of Chapter 6 to this issue, most educators will tell you these steps won't save a bad student or hurt a good one. The committee can get a pretty good picture of you as a candidate from your application, personal statement, and letters of recommendation. (The latter is the subject of its own chapter—number 11.)

Factors That Get You Noticed

Let's face it, if you have gotten this far in your career, you probably have the "smarts" to make the grade as a postgraduate trainee. (Resident, for those of you on the edges of that last statement.) That said, residency selection committees confront having to choose among a large number of fully qualified candidates. Your job is to stand out, rise above the crowd, be different, be better, faster, and wiser—in short, be noticed. Be your own best advocate and spokesperson.

Although you will probably use an electronic form of application for most residencies, a well-prepared, fully proofread, neatly presented personal résumé (the curriculum vitae, or CV) can be a real asset. This is so important that we will devote an entire chapter to the development of this lifelong tool.

A good CV and strong letters of recommendation are your best allies. But they will not be of much help if there is no content to work with. For this reason, early in the process you should look at yourself—who you are, where you have been, where do you want to go? This assessment should focus on activities and accomplishments. What have you racked up or what are logical undertakings to tackle at this stage of your career? Are there aspects of your personal growth and development that make you proud? Are there projects you meant to do but had put off? If they are logical at this stage of your life and you undertake them for their own sake (not just the application), now may be the time to do them. They may be a hobby, a talent, or an avocation. Become a youth leader, take up needlepoint, perfect you poetry, or charm a snake. These special things help set you apart. They are what make you interesting. They can also save your sanity when stresses build up.

Because much of the content of your letters of recommendation come from experiences that take place during your clinical rotations, treat each rotation as a prolonged interview. Your dress, demeanor, work ethic, punctuality, curiosity, and many other attributes will be out there for all to see. Is there something that you can find to do each day that will make you a better person, help someone else, or challenge you in some way? Are you living the ideals you want for yourself or are a part of your chosen field? Get to know your teachers, mentors, and members of the departments in which you rotate. They are the ones who will speak on your behalf to the selection committees through their letters of recommendation. The selection committees value this type of first-hand contact with candidates.

How They Carry Out the Process

Residency programs determine who they want on their lists through a very similar process to the one you are going through. No, they do not have to decide what type of candidate they want or what area of the country they want to teach in, but they do periodically reassess who they are and what goals they want to achieve. They decide (actively or passively) their balance among academic practical, service, teaching, and research. In part, they decide on what candidates they are looking for based on the previous experience of the program and the pool of candidates available in a given year. These factors work to your advantage in choosing programs. A program that in the past has been highly competitive (attracting the top of the class only) will probably be selective in the future. A program that sees itself as a stepping stone to subspecialty training and fellowships will be looking for like-minded students. These characteristics can help you refine your choices, ensuring the best match between you and your training program.

The program director, and sometimes others, will review the applications of candidates as they are received and make a preliminary determination about the appropriateness of an interview. This decision will revolve around a number of factors, including your basic science grades, performance on your clinical rotations, and board scores. Interview dates are established and some candidates are invited to schedule a visit. Spaces are left for qualified candidates who call to request a visit as well. The number of interview slots will vary from program to program, but there are often as many as ten to twenty interview slots for every position available.

Interview formats take as many forms as there are programs. The intent of the interview in all of its forms is to learn about you as a person. It is here that members of the department and selection committee develop a feel for your style, likes, dislikes, and character. This process is so vital to your success, that in Chapter 12 we will explore the process in detail.

Once the interview is over, some form of caucus takes place in which everyone who encountered the candidate has a chance to share his or her observations. This will include not only those who were part of the formal interview team, but also members of the department who were less apparent participants in the process. These may include the residents who gave the tour or those who took the candidates to lunch. This should alert you to be on your best behavior for the entire process. In this caucus, the candidates are given some form of ranking score that varies from program to program. Whether it is a 100-point scale or a letter grade, this is designed to help compare the students when the interview process ends, sometimes months later.

As the date to submit the final program ranking list approaches, there is often a final caucus involving the entire faculty and residents. Here a final review takes place. The student's portfolio is evaluated again and comparisons of the scores given earlier are made. This is where adjustments are made and people moved around on the list. Follow-up from the students, experience with them during a rotation, and other factors result in the students being bumped up or down in the rank order. Some of these factors you can control and are discussed in detail in Chapters 12 and 13. In most programs, the chairman or residency director reserves the right to determine the final list, though it will seldom be very different from the list developed in conjunction with the members of the department. The final list is almost always confidential.

The final list is determined by the perceived desirability of the candidates, not necessarily on the likelihood of an automatic match. Once the list is filed, the programs have to hold their breath just like the students do, waiting to see if they will fill their positions and their first choices. Just as with your list, if they place a name on the list, they have implicitly said that they would be happy to have the candidate join them as a resident no matter what their order on the list. For this reason, most programs will not publicize, not even to their own members, how far down the list a matching took place. It does not matter and most places won't tell you.

Chapter 4
The Master Timetable

Do you remember when you thought that next year would be less hectic and you would have more time? It didn't happen, did it? As life moves at the speed of a modem, you have to get organized or risk missing critical deadlines and pulling all-nighters to get your personal statement ready. Advanced planning not only will make life smoother but will give the look of an organized, reliable candidate—a definite plus. All you have to do is keep in mind what has to be done and create a timetable to keep you on track.

What Has to Be Done?

In the simplest form, the tasks are few: Pick a field of study and find programs of interest, fill out and file the applications, get letters of recommendation (and a dean's letter), interview, file your rank order list, wait, wait, wait, and celebrate. We have already looked at the issues of picking fields of study and how to begin to think about specific programs. Because it takes place part way into the process, the actual application form is the subject of a later chapter.

While we will look at the details of letters of recommendation later, they should be on your list of things to be thinking about from nearly the start of the process. Keep a list of faculty members who you work with who are possible resources for recommendations. This will prevent your forgetting an essential name when the time comes. Early in the year, feel free to ask prospective letter writers if they would be willing to give you a recommendation. If you decide to use them later, you have laid the groundwork; if you decide not to use them, they will have forgotten or they will be grateful that you did not need them.

To keep track of all the tasks involved, some form or database system should be seriously considered. Depending on your style and technical prowess, this may take the form of a card file, a three-ring binder, or computer database system (Figure 4-1). Even if you use the electronic application system (ERAS), there are still lots of details to be juggled, and a system will keep you from having something drop through the cracks. You will also want some sort of system to keep track of your impressions and observations when you come back from interviews. This is a time when all the hospitals in the country begin to look the same and only notations will save you.

Application / Inquiry Checklist
Program Name: _____
Program Director: _____
(Contact person): _____
Address: _____
City, State, Zip code: _____
Phone: _____ Fax: _____ e-mail: _____

		Date			
		Requested	Received	Sent	Arrived
	Information				
ERAS: Yes○ No ○	Application				
	Transcript				
	Recomendation #1				
	Recomendation #2				
	Recomendation #3				

Interview: _____
(Date, time, place)

Figure 4-1 An application tracking system can be as simple as a sheet of paper or a card.

Milestones to Shoot for

Knowing what has be done and getting it accomplished on time are not the same. Just as you should use a database system to keep track of what has been sent, received, etc., some form of reminder calendar is wise. This will help you keep track of time and avoid last-minute rushes that are stressful and less efficient. One form of this is a master schedule of events (Figure 4-2). You must be aware that some advanced or specialty programs will have different timetables than the ones provided here. It is your responsibility to keep up with the specifics; this book can only be a guide.

Junior year January	Choose an advisor and have first meeting
Mid-March	Plan senior curriculum (including electives)
April	Agreement materials for the NRMP are sent to medical schools
Mid-June	Student agreement materials for the NRMP for independent applicants are available
June - July	Prepare preliminary list of programs and meet with your advisor to discuss them Request applications and get application photo taken
Senior year Mid-July	**Deadline:** NRMP must receive agreement materials from U.S. students; early specialty match materials also due
July	Request information from residencies on your list Begin a personal statement and .V
August	Develop a database, card file, or other method of tracking information and deadlines Review your personal statement and CV
September	Request letters of recommendation from faculty Review your personal statement and CV with your advisor Begin applications
Mid-September	The NRMP Directory of programs is posted on the Web Review your list of programs with your advisor
Mid-October	**Deadline:** Complete submission of applications (deadlines vary, so be careful) Make preliminary inquiries about interviews
Mid-November	**Deadline:** NRMP must receive agreement materials from independent and sponsored graduate applicants
November - January	Interview at programs; make notes to yourself
1st week in January	Programs must file final list of quotas and withdrawals. Check for any changes in the programs of interest.
Mid-January	Make and file your rank order list
Mid-February	**Deadline:** Rank order lists must be filed by both programs and individuals
Match day—3	Matched and unmatched information is released to applicants at 12:00 noon eastern standard time (EST)
Match day—2	Filled and unfilled results for individual programs are posted to the Web at 11:30 a.m. EST; locations of all unfilled positions are released to applicants at 12:00 noon EST; unmatched applicants may begin contacting unfilled programs at 12:00 noon EST
Match day	Match results are given out at 12:00 noon EST Match results are posted on the NRMP Web site at 1:00 p.m. EST
March to Mid-April	Letters of appointment or agreement are sent to the student and must be returned

Figure 4-2 The Master Timetable

As you create your master timetable, don't forget to include time for the support jobs and the schedules of others that are involved as well. You will need extra time with your advisor (to review lists, CVs, personal statements, and the like) and others. Be sure you have taken into account their availability. There is nothing worse than having to have your advisor-approved schedule of classes for next year in the dean's office by 5 p.m. and discovering that your advisor is giving a lecture in Bora Bora.

Periodically look at your master timetable. Plan. Just because an event is listed for next month doesn't mean that it has to be put off. This is especially important for the more creative or time-consuming chores such as personal statements, your curriculum vitae, or telephone calls. Give yourself a safety cushion of a few days for unexpected disasters such as unavailable computer terminals, postal holidays, or the lack of stamps. Add this time to the tasks you expect from others as well; the less control you have over a deadline, the more buffer you should add.

There are a number of systems you can use to remind yourself of upcoming tasks and deadlines. These can be as simple as a desk or wall calendar or as complex as a computer reminder system. Between these extremes are the daily planners so favored by hospital administrators. Unless you normally carry one of these around, tracking your progress through the residency application process probably does not demand this degree of obsession. (The same is true for the palm-top electronic organizers. These also suffer from the added problems of dead batteries and loss or theft.)

Chapter 5
Choosing an Advisor

You have decided the field you want to pursue and have begun to think about your chances of matching. You have a sense of what the steps are going to be and the timetable for them, but it all still seems daunting. This is where your residency advisor comes in. He or she will be the most useful tool you have at your disposal. It is your advisor who can act as a touchstone for your thoughts, point you in the right direction, and keep you on track for a match that is right for you. He or she provides moral support and is an endless source of information that is not readily available anywhere else. This person is different for any advisors you have had during medical school thus far; he or she will be a mentor. This mentor is specific and skilled in the process of getting you into the residency of your choice. Given the value of your advisor, how do you go about getting the right one and using him or her to best advantage?

What to Look For

There are a number of attributes to look for in the advisor you choose. First, you should choose a member of the field of study you want to pursue. While much of the advice you will need is independent of your field of study, it will take someone within your specialty to give you the nuances and inside view, you require. Only an insider will have the connections to know the latest information about programs around the country.

Connectivity comes from the second attribute that you should look for in an advisor—involvement. If your advisor is actively involved at the state, regional, or national level, he or she is more likely to know about changes, strengths, or weaknesses of programs outside of your city. Involvement also gives your advisor contacts in other institutions so that questions can be answered, inquiries made, and personal referrals given.

The next attribute you should look for is maturity. While junior faculty are often more accessible, you should seek an advisor who has had some experience counseling or being a part of your institution's selection process. This will give the advisor "seasoning" and practical experience that will keep his or her suggestions down to earth. The experience of having seen other candidates will help your advisor put your strengths and weaknesses in perspective so that you receive realistic guidance about the programs you should consider.

You will want your mentor to have character. Your advisor must act as a role model, be steadfast to help you through your insecurities, and be circumspect enough to honor your trust and confidences. You need to be able to trust him or her to act in your best interests. He or she must be flexible enough to meet your unique needs, while resolute in his or her commitment to keep you from making mistakes of judgment.

Lastly, look for a good "fit." You should choose an advisor who has a style and personality that is compatible with your own. If you have a laid-back, let it happen style, an old-school autocrat won't be a good match. (In this case, though, someone who can gently keep you on track may still be a good idea.) Your style and that of your advisor should be congruent even if they are not the same. You want your advisor to be able to balance the roles of taskmaster, confessor, critic, and cheerleader.

If you are unsure of whom to pick, ask senior students who are already in the process. They will be able to tell you how their advisor has functioned and what they have heard from other students. Check with the dean's office at your school. The dean knows who writes the best letters and has a commitment to education and students. Ask the residents you have worked with. They work more closely with the faculty and get to know them well. They can tell you whom they might choose.

Some schools have formal systems of advising while others do not. If your school has a formal advisor system, check with the educational coordinator and clerkship director for the department to see what their procedures are. Many times, they will have a list of possible advisors. They may be able to help match you up, trying to meet your needs while avoiding a disproportionate load on any one faculty member. (Good advising takes time.)

Some schools will assign advisors based on clinical specialty. If this is the case, meet with your assigned advisor early and assess his or her ability to be a good advisor for your needs. Most schools that use this approach will pick only advisors with a good record of accomplishment, but your needs may be special. If you and your assigned advisor hit it off, you're in business. If you don't feel that the chemistry, expertise, or personality is what you need, keep this advisor for the formalities, and seek your own mentor.

If your school does not have a formal system of advisors, you are not completely on your own. Check with the clerkship director, the department chairman, or residency program director to ask who has acted as an advisor in the past. Feel free to set up a trial interview: Make an appointment to ask some questions about residencies in your field of interest. If you like the interaction, you can ask him or her to be your advisor. If you were not impressed, at least you got some questions answered. The less structured the system, the earlier you will want to select your advisor since the good ones will quickly become overwhelmed and stop taking on new students.

What You Don't Need

There are individuals who seem, on the surface, as if they would be good advisors. Unfortunately, they may not be the best choice. Knowing who you don't want is also important in the selection process.

You don't necessarily want the department head. He or she has risen far in the field and is highly respected by others, but may have a habit of being out of town or in a meeting just when you have a deadline you forgot about until the last minute. Don't worry about missing out on these strengths. Many programs require letters of recommendation from the department head and few will write these without first meeting you. This is your opportunity to use his or her expertise, without being tied to him or her for the month-to-month advising you need.

You don't necessarily need an emeritus member of the department as your advisor. While these individuals have a wealth of clinical and educational experience, it may not be current. In addition, they may not be in the network of educators from other institutions, or may not be aware of the often-changing pattern of resident education, the electronic application process (if applicable), or the Internet resources that are a part of the modern match.

You don't want to choose the residents and fellows you spent those long hours working with during your clerkship. While they know you well, they will lack the political clout to write letters and help get you interviews at your "gotta have it" institution. They can be good sources of informal advice, including whom to get as your advisor; they just are not it.

You don't want the world renowned-lecturers, book authors, or Nobel laureates. They are going to be too busy to be accessible. There are certainly exceptions, but be careful.

Do not choose someone who seems inflexible. The choices you have to make will be yours and only yours. Your advisor is just that, an advisor only. His or her role is to guide you in your choices. No one who wants to impose his or her thoughts on you has your best interests in mind. That is not to say that your advisor should not be forceful in keeping you on task and away from catastrophes, but he or she should recognize that ultimately the decisions are yours.

Using Them Wisely

Perfect advisors are of little use if you don't take advantage of them. There are a number of simple tricks that will ensure you get the most out of the advisor you have chosen.

Meet early and often; be visible. You should meet with your advisor early in the process. This "get-acquainted" visit will get the ball rolling. This familiarizes him or her with you and any special needs you might have. Your advisor must get to know you to be an effective mentor. Your mentor will often write letters of recommendation, or in some cases the body of your dean's letter, so he or she must know you on a personal basis. This early visit will allow you both to set out some target dates for milestones, should there be special circumstances that make them different from the norm. Your advisor can tell you of his or her preferences for appointments, drop-ins, telephone calls, and other access issues, and can tell you about travel scheduled around the time of major events in the matching process. This will make for fewer last-minute surprises should a deadline sneak up on you.

Do the legwork. When you meet with your advisor, plan ahead. Come prepared with information, questions, or requests. Be sure to provide your advisor with any information sufficiently in advance for him or her to act on it. If you want an opinion on your personal statement or CV (and you should), supply it well in advance of your meeting so your advisor has time to go over it. If you need information about a list of programs, get it to your advisor early. This will save those awkward moments when you sit looking decorative while your advisor goes over the paperwork.

Keep your advisor posted. Let your advisor know about your thoughts and plans. Talk over your preliminary list of programs early and often. When you get ready to go for an interview, let your advisor know. A call from your mentor to an old friend can mean a more personal welcome along the way. Give your advisor feedback when you return. This feedback is a good source of information for those advisees who follow you.

Do your homework. Don't expect your advisor to do your work for you. You will have to be the one who develops a list of possible programs. You are the one who has to request materials, complete filing procedures, and meet deadlines. Your advisor may be able to keep you on track, but it is your responsibility. Your advisor's value to you comes from his or her knowledge, expertise, connections, and experience, not secretarial or telephone skills.

Make your advisor work for you. Ask him or her to walk you through a mock interview. Ask for specific suggestions on your personal statement, not just general impressions. (This should not include grammar or spelling; that is your job.) Ask your advisor to suggest other programs you haven't considered. It is a rare advisor who will voluntarily share all the tricks and expertise he or she has without being asked.

Lastly, make friends with the support staff. Alienating your advisor's secretary and the clerkship coordinator is a sure way to kill access to them. Make enemies of these people and you may never see your advisor again except in the halls. (Your advisor may never even know it has happened.) These support people are the ones who can fit you in at the last minute, wangle that special favor, or get you the out-of-town hotel number where your advisor is staying when your world is falling apart. But do not expect them to place calls, write personal letters, request applications, or drop something in the mail for you; you can do these things yourself.

Chapter 6
Tryouts and Electives

As if life was not complicated enough, in the midst of beginning your search for the ideal residency, you still have to finish medical school. One part of that task will be the selection of senior electives. While the number and latitude of electives available will vary from school to school, the choice of electives cannot be treated lightly. The choices you make will affect not only your knowledge base but may be used to enhance your preparation for a residency. This is also a good opportunity to seek guidance from your mentor throughout this process.

Choosing Senior Electives

There is a tendency for students to focus on their field of interest when choosing electives. This is natural. You enjoy your chosen field and are anxious to get right into it. This, however, is not the best course to follow. Indeed, many specialties will only allow a limited senior experience in their own area, stressing a more balanced approach. There are, however, very valid reasons to obtain some additional experience in you field, but it should be balanced and timed so you get the maximum benefit.

Many students believe that additional experience in their chosen field will make them more attractive when they interview at prospective residencies. Residency selection committees look for a well-rounded background in their candidates. They know that in the years spent in residency training you will receive all the specialty experience you need. Two or three months of a senior elective will not make any difference in the end. Therefore, this extra course does not make you a more attractive candidate.

Some students want to do a senior elective in their chosen field to cultivate possible references and letters of recommendation. If your original rotation was at an affiliated institution, you may not be well known to the key people in your department. An elective at the main campus can help solve this. If you go this route, the elective must be taken no later than September of your senior year to allow time for letters to be written. This is also why you should not take time off between your junior and senior year: this is the last chance to get grades on the transcript that accompanies your application for a residency.

Some students see an additional rotation in their chosen field as a way to improve on a poor performance as a junior or to buttress an average transcript. This can only work if the elective is early enough in the year to make it onto the transcript by the time your application is filed. Let's be honest, if your performance was marginal as a junior, even an honors as a senior will not erase the taint. You need to be realistic about that, and plan your application strategies accordingly. This is where a good advisor will be critical to assess the damage and give you guidance.

How, then, should you go about choosing electives? The bulk of the core material you will need in your individual field of study will be provided in the residency. Consequently, look for ways to augment your background. Choose electives that will be useful, but unlikely, components of specialty training. For example, if you are going into a primary care field, consider additional experience in dermatology, emergency medicine, or pediatrics. If you are moving toward a surgical specialty, consider training in radiology, critical care, emergency medicine, or anesthesiology. If your field is a narrow one, consider additional time in general or family medicine. If your field has a strong research component or expectation, brush up on a basic science. Course work in anatomy, anatomic pathology, ethics, medicolegal issues, or the business of medicine is always useful.

Elective courses can also be ways of solidifying your career choice. Additional time in your chosen field can reinforce the correctness of your decision. Time spent in your second choice can remind you of why you did not make that choice; if your decision between two fields is a close one, this may be a wise course of action. It is better to make a change in career direction in the fall of your senior year than in the second or third year of residency. If you go this route, take the elective as the first or second one of the year. This allows for regrouping, if needed.

You may choose to take an elective to take advantage of a special opportunity. It might be a chance to study with a legendary figure, see cases of a type that are unique, or participate in a special program. It might be an elective that isn't offered anywhere else or at any other time.

Some students choose to take time off to study for the board examination, or to travel to interviews. This is a luxury not every student has available. For the most part, if you are not prepared for boards, a month of cramming will not materially change your chances of success. Since you will not know your interview schedule by the time you must register your electives (generally in the spring of your junior year), it is impractical to protect all of the time you might need for travel. For this reason, you might want to choose clerkships that will be tolerant of occasional departures for interview trips. When the time comes, don't abuse the good graces of the service to which you are assigned. Ask in advance and spread your travels over several rotations.

Some students like to lighten their load toward the end of their senior year to decompress after the match, to reduce burn out, or prepare for their move to residency. This is nice if you can do it, but remember that residency selection committees will often ask about the electives you plan. A curriculum that appears as if you are coasting suggests you might do the same as a resident.

Before you plan your senior year, check with your dean's office to see what requirements must be met. Many schools have guidelines for the types of course that must be included. You should also check with your advisor early in the process for more specific suggestions as well.

Electives as "Wild Hairs"

Electives do not always have to be of the "type A," goal-oriented, straight-laced type. Have you considered ways to expand your horizons? This is a time to think horizontally; to get out of the box (or out of Dodge, as the case may be). These are, after all, electives. If your school allows it, have you considered courses in business, the arts, economics, or basic sciences? Certainly, your entire senior year can't be made up of such courses, but some exposure to these options should be considered.

Some of your elective time can be spent (again, with the permission of your school) in other forms of personal growth. This could be experience as a medical missionary, work in a research laboratory, as a legislative assistant, or an opportunity to study the medical system of another country. You could pursue some lifelong interest. I know of one student who spent some of his elective time taking theater and performance courses at the graduate level.

The message here is: Think creatively. Do be aware that many programs and application forms will ask about the electives you have planned or have carried out. You must be able to justify and discuss your reasoning. Your choices, therefore, should challenge, stretch, and expand your horizons. An innovative choice can not only be fun, it can demonstrate your individuality and style.

Electives as Interviews

There is a great deal of debate about using electives as an extended interview. This form of elective is one taken in your chosen field and located in your most desired institution. The logic is that you will have an opportunity to be a part of the department on a day-to-day basis, demonstrating your qualifications. You have a chance to get to know the department members and they get a chance to know you. When it comes time to rank you, you are no longer a stranger, met just once months ago.

The idea is beguiling, but it is not all that simple. First, not all programs will offer electives to outside students, and not all schools will extend credit for this outside experience. You will be competing against the school's own students, potentially limiting the experience you get. You will have the trouble and expense of living away from your normal base of operations, requiring the logistics of finding housing, transportation, and so forth.

If you are willing to overcome the logistical obstacles, you need to keep in mind several other considerations. A prolonged interview in the form of an elective cannot overcome a bad transcript or board scores. While a good performance can speak on your behalf, a less than stellar performance can even hurt your chances. In the end, if you are a good student you probably don't need it, and if you are marginal it could even hurt you.

The consensus of most program directors seems to be that the interview elective will generally not make a big difference either way. Therefore, if the elective makes sense for other reasons (it is near home, offers extraordinary experiences, provides a chance to meet a luminary or work in a different environment), then take it. Otherwise, you can probably use the time more effectively in other ways. As with so much of the matching process, check with your advisor. See if he or she thinks you come across better in person or on paper. He or she can also look at your overall package and judge the value the rotation could have for you.

If you choose to do an out-of-town elective, avoid the months of November and December. During these months faculty members and residents take vacations, clinic schedules are reduced, and surgical loads are light. Write to the program of interest early because any available slots will fill fast. If slots are filled, you can consider a rotation in an allied field that might still give you exposure to members of your department of interest. While you are at the institution, make appointments to meet the essential members of the department. Don't forget to go to any conferences, grand rounds, or teaching programs offered by the department; they are good experience and show your commitment and initiative.

Chapter 7
Making the List—Your First Cut

The time has come to make your preliminary list of residencies. This is a working document that you will review and revise many times over the next few months. At this stage, it should be long and unfocused. It will include programs located near your medical school and programs far away. It should have highly competitive dream programs, intermediate ones, and some generally overlooked options as well. This list will be your first cut, but not your last. This is the list you will use to gather information, request brochures, and submit applications.

To establish this list, you need some sense of what is available. In Chapter 2, we looked at some of the factors that go into your choice of specialty, specialty options, location, and possible programs. Through this process, you probably know some programs to consider or know others by reputation, experience, or the advice of your advisor. While these options must be seriously considered, you will not want to limit your horizons at this stage. You can locate other programs to consider, and the information you need about them, from a number of sources.

Publications

A traditional source of information about residency programs is the *NRMP Directory* published each year by the National Residency Matching Program. (As of the 2000 match, the book is no longer printed in hard copy. Your dean's office, library, or advisor may have back copies of this or you may see the current version on the World Wide Web.) This list contains all of the programs that participate in the annual match process. While not all programs participate, this list is effectively complete, omitting less than 2% of residencies. The lists are arranged by state and by specialty (Figure 7-1). The listing includes the program's code number for the NRMP match, its type (categorical, preliminary, and specialty), and the program's quota of residents for the match. In the geographic listing, information is also provided about any affiliation the program has with a Accreditation Council for Graduate Medical Education (ACGME) accredited medical school (Figure 7-2). A mailing address and telephone number for the institution is provided, but not the specifics of the program director or department chairman.

```
┌─────────────────────────────────────────────────────────────────┐
│  2000 NRMP          NATIONAL RESIDENT                            │
│  Directory          MATCHING PROGRAM                            │
│  ─────────────────────────────────────────────────────────────  │
│              [ NRMP Home ]  [ AAMC Home ]                        │
│                                                                  │
│  ANESTHESIOLOGY                                                  │
│                                                                  │
│  ALABAMA                                                         │
│  Hospital Name              Code Type Quota                      │
│  U ALABAMA HSP-BIRMINGHAM   100751  S    14                      │
│                                                                  │
│  ARIZONA                                                         │
│  Hospital Name              Code Type Quota                      │
│  UNIV ARIZONA AFFIL HOSPS   101551  S     7                      │
│                                                                  │
│  ARKANSAS                                                        │
│  Hospital Name              Code Type Quota                      │
│  U ARKANSAS-LITTLE ROCK     101831  C     8                      │
│                                                                  │
│  CALIFORNIA                                                      │
│  Hospital Name              Code Type Quota                      │
│  LOMA LINDA UNIVERSITY-CA   102451  S    10                      │
│  U SOUTHERN CALIFORNIA      103351  S    10                      │
│  UCLA MEDICAL CENTER-CA     195651  S    15                      │
│  UC IRVINE MED CTR-CA       104351  S     5                      │
│  UC DAVIS MED CTR-SAC-CA    104651  S     8                      │
│                             104679  P     4                      │
│  UC SAN DIEGO MED CTR-CA    104951  S     8                      │
│  UC SAN FRANCISCO-CA        106251  S    20                      │
│  STANFORD UNIV PROGS-CA     182051  S    15                      │
│  HARBOR-UCLA MED CTR-CA     106731  C     2                      │
│                             106751  S     2                      │
│                                                                  │
│  COLORADO                                                        │
│  Hospital Name              Code Type Quota                      │
│  U COLORADO SOM-DENVER      107651  S    12                      │
│                                                                  │
│  CONNECTICUT                                                     │
│  Hospital Name              Code Type Quota                      │
│  UNIV OF CONNECTICUT        109451  S     8                      │
│                             109496  R     6                      │
│  YALE-NEW HAVEN HOSP-CT     108951  S     6                      │
│                                                                  │
│  DISTRICT OF COLUMBIA                                            │
│  Hospital Name              Code Type Quota                      │
│  GEORGE WASHINGTON U-DC     180251  S     7                      │
└─────────────────────────────────────────────────────────────────┘
```

Figure 7-1 This is an example of the specialty listing for programs participating in the NRMP match. (Reprinted with permission from the National Resident Matching Program, 1999.)

```
┌─────────────────────────────────────────────────────────────────────┐
│  2000 NRMP        NATIONAL RESIDENT                                   │
│  Directory        MATCHING PROGRAM                                    │
│  ─────────────────────────────────────────────────────────────────   │
│              ┌─────────────┐ ┌─────────────┐                         │
│              │  NRMP Home  │ │  AAMC Home  │                         │
│              └─────────────┘ └─────────────┘                         │
│                Hospitals are listed alphabetically by city.           │
│  WYOMING                                                              │
│                                                                       │
│  UNIVERSITY OF WYOMING-CASPER                                         │
│  FAMILY PRACTICE-CASPER                                               │
│  1522 EAST A ST                                                       │
│  CASPER, WY 82601                                                     │
│  Telephone:  (307) 266-3076                                           │
│      Association: NO ASSOCIATIONS                                     │
│         Program Description         Code   Type  Quota                │
│         FAMILY PRACTICE C           308920  C     8                   │
│  UNIV OF WYOMING-CHEYENNE                                             │
│  821 E 18TH ST                                                        │
│  CHEYENNE, WY 82001-4775                                             │
│  Telephone:  (307) 777-7911                                           │
│      Association: NO ASSOCIATIONS                                     │
│         Program Description         Code   Type  Quota                │
│         FAMILY PRACTICE C           203420  C     6                   │
└─────────────────────────────────────────────────────────────────────┘
```

Figure 7-2 This is an example of the geographic listing for programs participating in the NRMP match. (Reprinted with permission from the National Resident Matching Program, 1999.)

Students interested in residency programs located in Canada can find information at the Canadian Residency Matching Program's Web site (http://www.carms.ca/director.htm, Figure 7-3). This Web page includes far more information about salaries, leave times, and other benefits than do the pages available from the NRMP or the American Medical Association (shown below). This is because of the smaller number of programs (thirteen) available in Canada.

CaRMS Program Directory
1999-2000

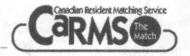

Please read this introduction

The *CaRMS Program Directory* is an up-to-date listing of postgraduate programs available at 13 of the 16 Canadian medical schools. It is revised frequently as programs are updated, requirements change and other new information is sent to CaRMS by the various medical schools across Canada.

Because students applying for postgraduate positions depend on the information listed in the *CaRMS Directory* , beginning in September, changes are announced in the newsletter, *Applying To You* , and highlighted in the program indices with the following symbols:
[UPDATED]   [NEW]

Please also take note of the last date of revision of a program description at the bottom of each program page.

Indices for Programs

 Programs by specialty,

including an option to print mailing labels by specialty .

 Programs by university

 Programs offering positions, but not through CaRMS

Figure 7-3 The Canadian Residency Matching Program (CaRMS) maintains a Web site that lists residency slots available in Canada. (Reprinted with permission from the Canadian Residency Matching Program, 1999.)

Some programs in the NRMS listing carry a special designation ("+") following their quota of positions offered. These programs differ from the majority that have a fixed resident compement. These programs may have their quota increased through a procedure that occurs during the matching process called reversion. Reversion of positions occurs if another program in the same institution (or group of institutions) does not fill its quota through the normal match process. A designated number of the unfilled positions then revert to the receiving program, increasing its quota. This most often occurs for programs in internal medicine, family medicine, and general pediatrics when a more specialized path in these areas at the same institution does not fill. If you are considering a program that may receive slots by reversion, you are safest to assume that you are competing for the minimum number. Don't count on extra places to magically appear.

One hint: when you are looking for possible programs based on locations and the city of interest is near a state border or part of a metropolitan area, look in the adjacent areas as well. Many times, a very good program may be located only blocks away across a border or city boundary, thus giving it a different listing. So, if you are looking at programs in Baltimore, check out Washington, D.C. as well. If you were to check Kansas City, Missouri, you should include Kansas City, Kansas, as well, and so on.

The Internet

There is a wealth of information available on the Internet regarding residency programs, the application process, and the match. Through Internet sites, you can find lists of programs in most specialties and specific information about many programs. The best sources of information about residencies and hospitals are sites maintained by the American Medical Association (AMA) and the Association of American Medical Colleges (AAMC).

The AMA maintains a site known as FREIDA (Fellowship and Residency Electronic Interactive Database). This site contains a large amount of information about hospitals and programs in the United States (Figure 7-4). Links contained in this site will lead the user to various pieces of information including work force assessments, the duration of training, and even resident work hours.

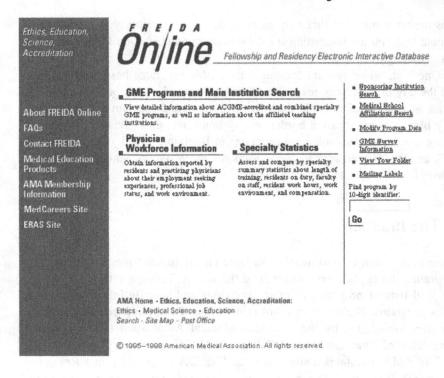

Figure 7-4 The URL for FREIDA online is:

http://www.ama-assn.org/cgi-bin/freida/freida.cgi.

A useful feature of this site is the ability to look up information about particular programs and institutions (Figure 7-5). The site not only provides information about the hospital (Figure 7-6) but also gives links to information about the community that may be helpful in considering a residency option (Figure 7-7).

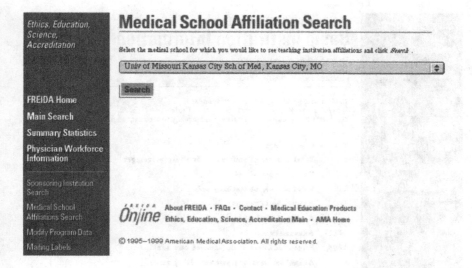

Figure 7-5

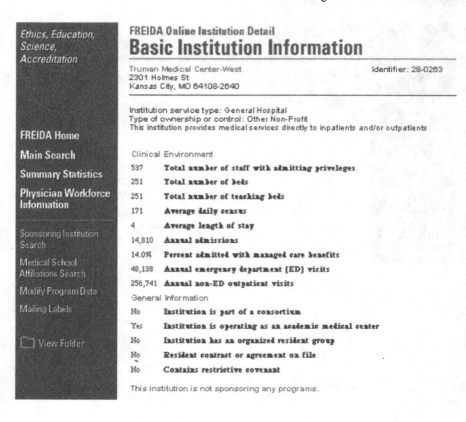

Figure 7-6

Expanded Institution Information

- Special Clinical Resources
- Sources of Payment
- Major Medical Benefits
- Community Data

- Medical School Affiliation
- Affiliated Program List
- View All Institution Info

Figure 7-7

The AAMC is the moving force behind the Electronic Residency Application Service (ERAS) Web site that contains information about programs that participate in the electronic application process (Figure 7-8). This site contains information about the electronic application process but also has links to information about specific programs (Figure 7-9). Through this resource, programs in specific specialties are listed geographically (Figure 7-10). This may give you ideas about regional programs that you may have overlooked.

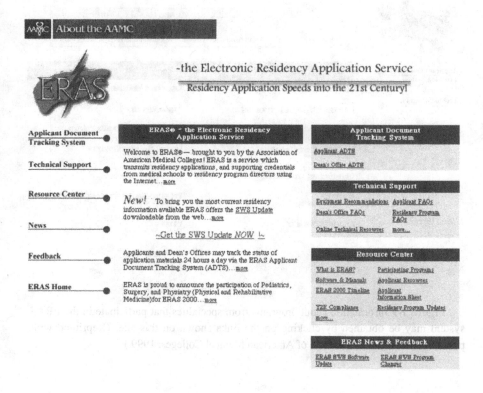

Figure 7-8 The American Association of Medical Colleges maintains the ERAS site. (Reprinted with permission from the Association of American Medical Colleges, 1999.)

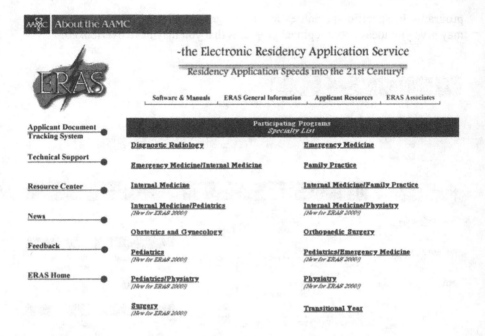

Figure 7-9 Information about programs from specialties that participate in the ERAS system may be obtained by clicking on the links shown on this site. (Reprinted with permission from the Association of American Medical Colleges, 1999.)

ERAS 2000 Participating Programs
Obstetrics & Gynecology

- Applicants are advised to contact each residency program for definitive information about the residency program's accreditation status, requirements, and deadlines **before** submitting any application materials.
- ERAS is not an authority on accreditation and is not responsible for any changes in a residency program's status after our software has been finalized.

The list is ordered by state, then city, then residency program name.

Programs in grey/italics are not participating in ERAS 2000

	Obstetrics & Gynecology	
2200111018	University of Alabama Medical Center Program	Birmingham, AL
2200121020	University of South Alabama Program	Mobile, AL
2200411026	University of Arkansas for Medical Sciences Program	Little Rock, AR
2200321024	Good Samaritan Regional Medical Center Program	Phoenix, AZ
2200321328	Phoenix Integrated Residency Program in Obstetrics and Gynecology	Phoenix, AZ
2200321025	University of Arizona Program	Tucson, AZ
2200531027	Kern Medical Center Program	Bakersfield, CA
2200531029	University of California (San Francisco)/Fresno Program	Fresno, CA
2200531030	Glendale Adventist Medical Center Program	Glendale, CA
2200521329	Loma Linda University Program	Loma Linda, CA
2200531034	Cedars-Sinai Medical Center Program	Los Angeles, CA
2200521037	Charles R Drew University Program	Los Angeles, CA
2200511036	Los Angeles County and University of Southern California Program	Los Angeles, CA
2200512035	Southern California Kaiser Permanente Medical Care (Los Angeles) Program	Los Angeles, CA
2200531038	UCLA Medical Center Program	Los Angeles, CA
2200521039	White Memorial Medical Center Program	Los Angeles, CA
2200512040	Kaiser Permanente Medical Group (Oakland) Northern California Program	Oakland, CA
2200521031	University of California (Irvine) Program	Orange, CA
2200521028	University of California (Davis) Program	Sacramento, CA
2200511012	Naval Medical Center (San Diego) Program	San Diego, CA
2200521044	University of California (San Diego) Program	San Diego, CA
2200512045	Kaiser Permanente Medical Group (San Francisco) Northern California Program	San Francisco, CA
2200521047	University of California (San Francisco) Program	San Francisco, CA
2200521333	Santa Clara Valley Medical Center Program	San Jose, CA
2200512311	Kaiser Permanente Medical Group (Santa Clara) Northern California Program	Santa Clara, CA
2200521048	Stanford University Program	Stanford, CA
2200521050	Los Angeles County-Harbor-UCLA Medical Center Program	Torrance, CA

Figure 7-10 This is a partial example of the program listing for obstetrics and gynecology available through the ERAS site. This is representative of the type of listing available for other specialties as well. (Reprinted with permission from the Association of American Medical Colleges, 1999.)

One drawback to this listing is that you cannot directly access further information about the program from this site. However, you can use the information gained to look up information from other sites, including FREIDA.

A large number of institutions and individual programs now have Web sites of their own. These sites highlight their institution and program, often containing as much or more information than a traditional brochure (Figure 7-11). At most of these sites, you can click on links within the page to be taken to more information. Web site information is not limited to the big university-based programs or specialty pursuits (Figures 7-12 and 7-13).

The Residency Brochure

Chairman's Welcome
Philosophy & Goals
Residency & Medical Center History
About the Department of Emergency Medicine
Residency Curriculum
Residency Didactic Program
Applications, Selection Procedure, and Student Elective Rotations
Chairman's Summary
DEM Home Page

Chairman's Welcome

Dear Colleagues:

This residency web site is a brief presentation of the **strongest training program** for physicians choosing to specialize in Emergency Medicine, the newest primary specialty.

The **residency program** here at LAC+USC Medical Center is the **largest and one of the oldest programs nationally**. The Department of Emergency Medicine at this medical center was the **first free-standing academic Department of Emergency Medicine in the country**. Since its' inception in 1971, over 400 physicians have graduated from this pioneering program.

The most significant evaluation of a training program is the competence and quality of its' graduates. Upon completion of this program, you will be fit and proud to join those who have gone before you. Together you will feel competent and comfortable managing the most difficult cases presenting to any Emergency Department in the nation.

Gail V. Anderson,MD FACEP
Professor and Chairman
Department of Emergency Medicine
LAC+USC Medical Center
Los Angeles, California 90033
(323) 226-6667

▲ Table of Contents

Figure 7-11 This is an example of an on-line residency brochure from the University of Southern California program in Emergency Medicine. Like most program sites, this one is long on information and short on modesty. Clickable links direct you to additional information.

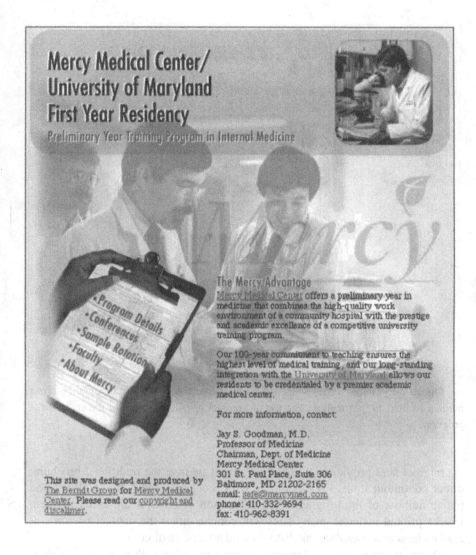

Figure 7-12 This is an example of an on-line residency brochure from a community program (with university affiliations). The program is a preliminary year in general medicine.

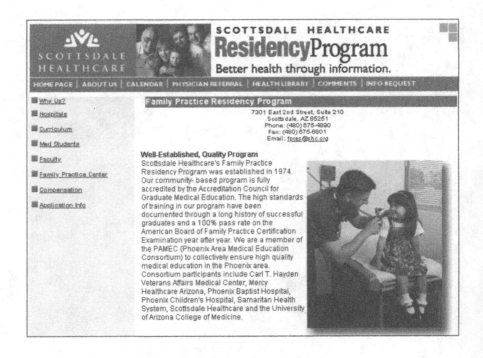

Figure 7-13 The Web site of this community-based family medicine program offers a number of links to information. The use of graphics provides a sense of the style of the program.

Internet sites provide one additional advantage over the traditional brochure: direct communications via e-mail. As with brochures, the name, address, and phone number of the program's contact person or director are usually given. Unlike printed material, many sites will contain either the contact person's e-mail address or a clickable link that will send a message directly.

Electronic mail is a rapid means of communicating with programs. With e-mail, you can keep one or more programs posted on your progress, request written materials, and follow up on interview dates. For example, most e-mail systems allow you to prepare a template that you can use like stationery: just electronically "tear off" a copy and send it. This can save time and allow you to send the same message repeatedly to different programs. Warning: if you address the message to more than one destination at the same time, each individual who gets the message will be able to see the names of everyone else receiving it at the same time. If you don't want to publicize your plans, send each message individually. The message can be the same, you just need to personalized the electronic "envelope" that has the address.

As the presence of residency Web sites, electronic application forms, and e-mail enough to justify or require Internet access? For most, the answer is yes. This does not mean that you have to string exotic phone lines to you home, purchase the latest notebook computer, and have your own personal Web site. If you have access through your medical school, that is more than adequate. Medical school libraries usually have Internet access for their users. These connections are generally faster than what you can get from home, and you can let someone else worry about the expense, maintenance, and hardware. If e-mail is not available at your institution, free e-mail hosting is available from a number of sites on the Internet.

Brochures

Paper brochures are the mainstays of residency information. Even residencies with electronic Web sites have paper versions of their information. Like Web sites these brochures give an overview of the program, its philosophy, rotations, call schedules, benefits, faculty lists, and other details. Printed pamphlets allow you to make a physical file that you can refer to, even when you are not near a computer.

Because these circulars contain slightly different information than do most Web sites, it is not a bad idea to request them as a supplement to what you already have. The simplest way to do this is by postcard (Figure 7-14). At this point in the process, a simple, but impersonal, approach is perfectly acceptable. Later, a more personal touch is wise. Since most programs still rely on a physical file for their residency applicants, the use of a postcard will begin a file, while an electronic request may not. In a similar way, the physical flier from the program will be a stronger prompt for you to begin developing a file as well. There is nothing wrong with either method of requesting information—both work and have their own advantages and disadvantages.

Dear Program Director:

    I am interested in residency positions in the field of *[blank]* and would appreciate further information about the program you offer. This information may be sent to me at the following address:

        Stellar Student
        123 Main Street
        Central City, AB, 09110

          Thank you for your assistance

Stellar Student

Figure 7-14 This is an example of simple postcard request for program information.

Experts

We have previously discussed the value of a good advisor. Here is yet another way you can take advantage of his or her experience: ask for suggestions of programs to be considered. You chose your advisor because he or she knew the field and was experienced in resident education. Now tap into that. Ask which programs would he or she look at if it were his or her choice? Which program would be recommended for a relative? Which programs are overlooked gems? Which programs are overrated? To maximize effectiveness, you should seek this advice at the very beginning of the process and then again as you start to receive information from your requests.

    Don't limit yourself to just your advisor when seeking expert opinions. Ask the residents you work with about other programs they considered before deciding on your institution. (Don't ask if this was their first choice; of course it was!) You can use this question as an entrée to meet with other faculty members, the program director, or the department chairman. Don't be afraid to cast your net widely. Remember that at this stage you are not obligated to put any of the suggestions you receive on your final list.

Fellow Students

While this last source of information is the most readily accessible, it is also of very limited value. It is a good idea to ask your fellow students about programs they have visited during the interview process. Unfortunately, that is still some time off and the tactic is better used to winnow programs rather than select them for initial consideration.

You can take advantage of the experience of those senior students with whom you interact. They have been through part or all of the process and may be able to tell you about programs they have considered or visited. Find out who is contemplating the same field that you are. If the match has already taken place, find out who is going into your field and where they are going. Seek these students out. They will most often be glad to share their experiences, both good and bad. (Some departments even hold get-togethers or luncheons after the match to let juniors and seniors going into their field interact. If your institution does this, take advantage of it, if for nothing else than the free food.)

No matter what sources you use, remember that this is your list and it is just a starting point. You are still *making* the list; it is not yet *the* list.

Chapter 8
Application Forms

In the past, the application process was a chaotic one with as many different forms, deadlines, and particulars as there were programs. Now, the process is much simpler with the Universal Application Form and the Electronic Residency Application Service (ERAS). The National Residency Matching Programs (NRMP) has also simplified things by providing a series of uniform dates for the process.

Despite the simplifications made, the onus is still on the applicant to do the work. Programs cannot and will not seek you out. You are responsible for the forms, the process, and the deadlines (some still vary from program to program). Time goes by fast and this is not the place for a missed deadline. Use those type-A skills that got you into medical school and get your material in early. The earlier your application is completed and submitted, the earlier you can nail down an interview. You get dates that fit better into your schedule and you don't get frozen out at the last minute because all the slots are taken.

Do remember that if you are applying to a program that requires a preliminary year, you may have to apply for both the preliminary and advance training positions at the same time. This situation may happen to applicants in many fields. Examples include anesthesia, emergency medicine, orthopedic surgery, and diagnostic radiology.

Paper or Plastic?

One decision you will not have to make for yourself is the choice between a paper application or the electronic equivalent, ERAS. [For some surgical subspecialties there is a comparable Central Application Service (CAS) that is discussed in greater detail in Chapter 15.] The specialty or program you choose will have made this decision for you. If your specialty has chosen to use the electronic system, almost every program within that specialty will follow suit. (Unfortunately, it is not 100%, so do check with each program individually to be sure.) The electronic application program allows for uniformity, and speed and reduces mailing costs, but substitutes some restrictions on individuality and adds escalating fees based on the number of programs you apply to. The current application fees (for July 1999 to June 2000) are $60 for up to ten programs; eleven to twenty programs, $6 each; twenty-one to thirty programs, $12 each; above thirty programs, $25 each. (Don't let this keep you from applying to a comfortable number of programs, though.) Programs that use the electronic application may also request the submission of a hard copy or the completion of an institutional application as well. (This is becoming less common as experience with the electronic version grows.)

The mainstay of the application process has always been the paper application. The NRMP makes available a paper Universal Application for Residency form (Figure 8-1). A Portable Document Format (PDF) version of this form is available on the Internet and paper copies are sent to the dean's office of each school. This form may be copied and used for most residency programs, though there are a few that will request additional information or require completion of their own form. Again, check with the individual program to be sure. As paper forms disappear, this is becoming less of a problem. Note: if a program gives you the choice between its form and the universal application, use its form. It shows a greater degree of interest and commitment to the individual program.

If your residency application is going to be paper based, remember the main rule: neatness counts—big time. This is a job application and so it must look and be professional. Whether you use the universal application or one specific for a given program, you will need several blank copies to work with. Therefore, the first task is to make several high-quality photocopies of the *blank* form. Set the original and two extra copies aside and protect them from folding, coffee spills, and misplacement. These are your backups, and there is a good chance you will need them.

Start by reading through the application. This is to ensure that you understand what is being requested and so you know where various types of information will be recorded. This read-through allows you to gather your thoughts about what facts you will need (dates of attendance, mailing addresses, etc.) and avoid the problem of putting information in the wrong place. If there are any questions, check with your dean's office, office of student affairs, or the residency itself. A simple mistake made because you didn't ask reflects badly on you and is easily avoided.

The second step is to fill in the blanks on a scratch copy. This can be in pencil, ink, or typing, because this will not be your final copy. See how the information fits. Will you need to use attachments to get it all in? Some applications allow attachments and some don't, so read the fine print. If you can avoid attachments without crowding or omitting critical information, do so. Since the people who will review your application have to look at lots of these documents, they are used to finding specific information in specific places. Using attachments breaks this rhythm. Don't shortchange yourself. If the only way to get vital information into your application (and have it readable) is to use an attachment, then use it. If you can use a smaller type, omit a low-priority item, or include it elsewhere in the application, then go that route. Remember the rule: neatness counts.

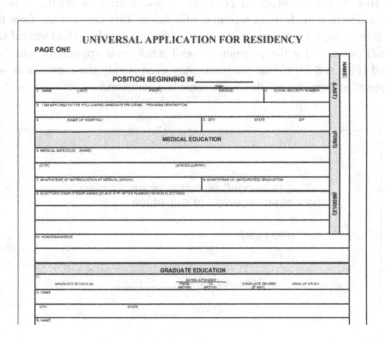

Figure 8-1 The Universal Application for Residency is made available by the National Residency Matching Program. (Reprinted with permission from the National Resident Matching Program, 1999.)

Once you think you have all the problems solved, it is time to fill in the blanks for real. This is best done on a typewriter[1] with fresh ribbon, preferably a carbon-film type. (Do check the directions: I know of one program that asked for a handwritten personal statement just to see if the applicants were reading the instructions.) Unless otherwise instructed, use a typewriter even if it means bribing a friend to do the job. Use clean hands to handle the form and do not use strikeovers or erasures. This is why you made so many copies earlier. Once it is completed, make a copy of the completed form. This copy serves two functions: you will want one for your records, and it is the copy that you share with a trusted friend to proofread. If any error is found, retype the entire page.

---

[1] There is no practical way to do this by computer at the present time. It is very probable that in the near future, this form may be downloaded, filled in electronically, and then printed, eliminating this step. Until then, you are stuck with trying to find a typewriter.

Remember that you will submit an original with an original signature to each program, not a copy.

Before you send in the finished application, reread the instructions for any enclosures that your program requires. If everything is ready, send the application with some form of receipt confirmation. This can take the form of a return receipt from the postal or courier service or a simple self-addressed (and stamped) postcard for the program to send when your application has been received (Figure 8-2). (Some programs may even supply these postcards with the application form, though this has become less common.)

This is to confirm that your application has been received in our office.

[Program]
[City]

Received by: _____

Date: _____

Figure 8-2 A self-addressed stamped card can serve to confirm receipt of your paper application packet.

Receipt of your application is not the same as having completed the application process. To verify that all the required materials have been received (such as letters of recommendation, transcripts, etc.) a more personal approach is in order. If you supply some form of mail-back card with your application, it is unlikely that the overworked staffers will think of sending it back to you when the last item arrives. Therefore, the only practical way to check on your application is to call. This provides positive confirmation, shows your interest, and helps make your name familiar to the office staff (not a bad thing). Don't wear out your welcome; make this call near the time interviews are to be scheduled and you are reasonably sure everything should have been received. This follow-up can be especially important if there is the possibility of items being incorrectly filed due to a name change or cultural confusion over which is a first or last name.

The ERAS System

In 1995-1996, the American Association of Medical Colleges (AAMC) introduced the Electronic Residency Application Service (ERAS). The system was first tested by residencies in obstetrics and gynecology and is now used by 16 specialties (Table 8-1), with more considering it. The ERAS system is composed of four components (software programs): the Student Workstation, the Dean's Office Workstation, the Program Directors Workstation, and the ERAS Post Office.

Table 8-1 Programs Participating in the ERAS Program for 1999 - 2000

Diagnostic radiology	Emergency medicine
Emergency medicine/Internal medicine	Family practice
Internal medicine	Internal medicine/Family practice
Internal medicine/Pediatrics	Internal medicine/Physiatry
Obstetrics and Gynecology	Orthopedic surgery
Pediatrics	Pediatrics/Emergency medicine
Pediatrics/Physiatry	Physiatry
Surgery	Transitional year

Ophthalmology, otolaryngology, neurosurgery, and plastic surgery use their own central application and matching services.

The Student Workstation Software (SWS) is installed on your computer so you can complete the process at home, at your own pace. This does require that you have a compatible computer (Table 8-2). If you do not have a computer, check to find out if the software is available in your library or dean's office. You can obtain the SWS from your dean's office, or from the Internet at:

http://www.aamc.org/eras/swsdisk/start.htm

This site offers the program in several formats that allow direct installation, delayed installation, or downloading to individual diskettes for installation on another machine. While you can install the software yourself through this method, you must obtain your Student Data Diskette directly from your dean's office (or other office designated at your school). Students who have already graduated from a United States medical school should consult the dean's office where they graduated. International medical graduates should contact the Educational Commission for Foreign Medical Graduates (ECFMG). Canadian medical graduates should contact the Canadian Resident Matching Service (CaRMS).

Table 8-2 Student Workstation Equipment Recommendations

Minimum Equipment	Recommended Equipment
486 PC-compatible computer capable of running Microsoft Windows 3.1	Pentium computer Microsoft Windows 95 or higher
8-MB RAM	16-MB RAM
3.5" floppy disk drive	3.5" floppy disk drive
A hard disk with 10 MB of file space	A hard disk with 40 MB of file space

ERAS Student Workstation Software (SWS) is not available as a Macintosh native application. If you can run other programs designed to run under Windows, you may be able to run the ERAS SWS. ERAS does not provide technical support for Macs, so you are somewhat on your own.

Using the SWS, you develop your application by filling in blanks and selecting from various options. Within the software, you also complete a program designation list indicating programs to which you want your application sent. The software then stores this information on a "Student Data Diskette." This diskette is then taken to the designated location at your school (most often the dean's office or office of student affairs). This office then submits the information to the ERAS post office by way of the Internet. The ERAS computers store the information for distribution to the individual residency programs. The individual residency program also receives the information by Internet connection, though it has to sign on and download the applications; they are not delivered automatically.

There are some minor differences in the procedure use by graduates of schools of osteopathy and foreign medical graduates. Osteopathic applicants apply directly through their medical schools, while graduates of foreign medical schools forward their diskettes and supporting documentation to the ECFMG. Canadian students forward ERAS application materials to the CaRMS.

Applications using the ERAS system offer several advantages over the older paper system. For one, you have to fill in the application form only once, and since it is electronic, you can retype it as many times as you wish without having to run to the copy machine. In addition, the system is faster and more efficient at filing and tracking your applications. ERAS offers a document tracking system that allows you to keep track of the status of the applications you submit. The ERAS Applicant Document Tracking System (ADTS) allows you or the dean's office to get a snapshot of the status of your documents. This report is based on activity as recently as the 24 hours before the request. With the ADTS you have the ability to check the arrival status of your application documents at selected programs. For security reasons, you need your user ID and password that was used to create your Student Workstation Diskette to access the information. One quirk of the system to be aware of: the passwords for your Student Data Diskette are not case sensitive, while they are for the ADTS, so be careful when you type.

With the ERAS system, you do not have to have all of your documents completed to begin the application process. You can submit your application form and personal statement, and have your letters of recommendation and dean's letter added later. (The dean's letter can be sent to the ERAS post office at any time, but it cannot be downloaded by the programs prior to 12 noon on November 1.) When additions to your application become available, the ERAS post office will update your application with each residency program when it next downloads information.

Like the paper application process, ERAS allows the applicant to customize the application you submit for each program. This allows you to specify which letters of recommendation go to which programs, to have different personal statements, and the like. This flexibility can be very useful. You can optimize your application to each program and your advisor can help you get the most out of this capability.

The ERAS system can be used to electronically submit copies of your USMLE scores. The National Board of Medical Examiners (NBME) is responsible for releasing the United Stated Medical Licensing Examination (USMLE) transcripts. In general, NBME will process an electronic request for transcripts within a few days of receiving a request from the ERAS post office. To have this information sent electronically, you must assign the USMLE transcript to the selected programs in the Assign Documents portion of the student workstation software. You will know if you have assigned the USMLE transcript correctly if the USMLE transcript appears in the "Documents Assigned to this Program" box. This transcript request will be sent to the NBME which processes the request and forward the electronic USMLE transcript to the selected programs. There is a $40 flat fee for requesting this transcript, but the fee covers the transmission of the information to all of your programs, regardless of the number you are applying to. If you choose, these transcripts can be automatically updated as your step II scores become available. Participating programs may request osteopathic students to send an electronic copy of their Comprehensive Osteopathic Medical Licensing Examination (COMLEX) or National Board of Osteopathic Medical Examiners (NBOME) transcript. Since ERAS only submits the USMLE electronically, you will have to submit this as a hard copy. (There are ways of scanning in the information so it comes out electronically, but they aren't worth the trouble; just mail it.)

Potential concerns about the ERAS system that are sometimes expressed are the issues of confidentiality and security. Access to the information in your application is only accessible by you, your dean's office, and the programs you designate. Your program selection list as well as the total number of programs you are applying to are confidential and are not seen by the residency programs you specify. This is also true of the number of letters of recommendation you have requested. Your dean's office does have access to this information because status reports that track all applicant documents transmitted from the dean's office are sent to it on a weekly basis by ERAS.

Remember there are costs associated with using the ERAS application. The sliding scale of fees (cited earlier in this chapter) has been used to discourage indiscriminant application to every program listed, the electronic equivalent of bulk mail. Graduates of foreign medical schools pay an additional handling fee to the ECFMG, for its service as the student's designated dean's office. As noted before, applicants who request USMLE transcripts via ERAS can send an unlimited number of electronic transcripts for a $40 fee to NBME or ECFMG.

Do keep an eye on the ERAS Internet Web site. This site will keep you informed about changes to programs that may be important to your application process (Figure 8-3). While most of these changes involve things like program name changes, it is wise to monitor the process. Also, remember that ERAS does not have any application deadlines; each individual program establishes its own deadlines. Schools may set deadlines regarding the transmission schedules and processing of letters of recommendation, but these are not the same as an application deadline, so check.

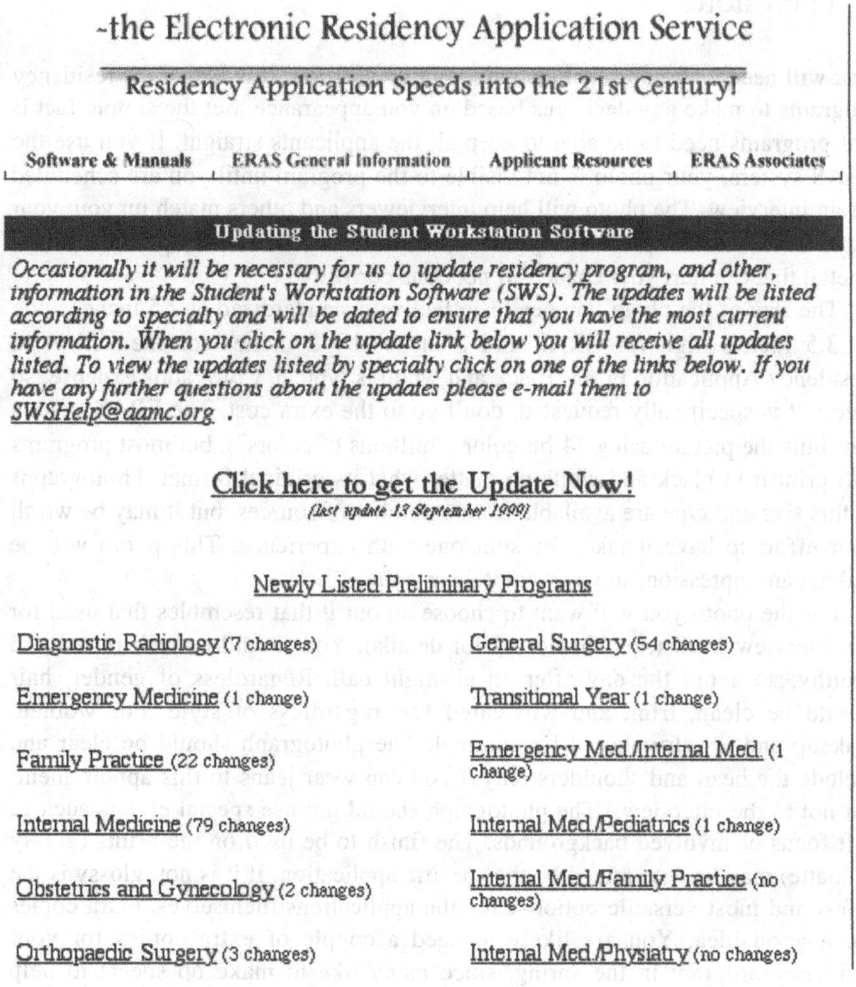

~the Electronic Residency Application Service

Residency Application Speeds into the 21st Century!

| Software & Manuals | ERAS General Information | Applicant Resources | ERAS Associates |

Updating the Student Workstation Software

Occasionally it will be necessary for us to update residency program, and other, information in the Student's Workstation Software (SWS). The updates will be listed according to specialty and will be dated to ensure that you have the most current information. When you click on the update link below you will receive all updates listed. To view the updates listed by specialty click on one of the links below. If you have any further questions about the updates please e-mail them to SWSHelp@aamc.org .

Click here to get the Update Now!

[last update 13 September 1999]

Newly Listed Preliminary Programs

Diagnostic Radiology (7 changes)

Emergency Medicine (1 change)

Family Practice (22 changes)

Internal Medicine (79 changes)

Obstetrics and Gynecology (2 changes)

Orthopaedic Surgery (3 changes)

General Surgery (54 changes)

Transitional Year (1 change)

Emergency Med./Internal Med. (1 change)

Internal Med./Pediatrics (1 change)

Internal Med./Family Practice (no changes)

Internal Med./Physiatry (no changes)

Figure 8-3 The ERAS update screen will tell you about changes in participating programs. (Reprinted with permission from the Association of American Medical Colleges, 1999.)

The Photo

You will need a photo to include with your application. It is illegal for residency programs to make any decisions based on you appearance, but the simple fact is that programs need to be able to keep all the applicants straight. If you use the ERAS system, your photo is not visible to the program until you are scheduled for an interview. The photo will help interviewers and others match up you, your paper work, and the person they remember. Like so much of the process, this is a detail that can hurt your chances if not done correctly.

The size of the photo you need is effectively standardized at 2.5 inches wide by 3.5 inches high for ERAS and 2 inches by 2 inches for the Universal Residency Application Form. Black and white is typical. Color adds expense, so unless it is specifically requested, don't go to the extra cost. The ERAS system transmits the picture using 24-bit color ("millions of colors"), but most programs will print it in black and white no matter what its original format. Photographs of this size and type are available from a number of sources, but it may be worth your effort to have it taken by someone with experience. This photo will be making an impression, so you want it done right.

For the photo you will want to choose an outfit that resembles that used for the interview itself (see Chapter 12 for details). You should be well rested and healthy, so avoid the day after an all-night call. Regardless of gender, hair should be clean, trim, and will cared for, regardless of style. For women, makeup and jewelry should be minimal. The photograph should be clear and include the head and shoulders only. (You can wear jeans to this appointment, but not to the interview.) The photograph should not use special effects such as soft focus or involved backgrounds. The finish to be used on the prints (glossy or matte) may be determined by the specific application. If it is not, glossy is the safest and most versatile option. Like the applications themselves, extra copies are a good idea. You are likely to need a couple of extra copies for your residency program in the spring, since many like to make up sheets to help identify the incoming house staff.

Chapter 9
The CV

Whether you use a paper application or an electronic one, one paper document you will want to prepare is your curriculum vitae or CV. You will use this document throughout your medical career for purposes as diverse as job applications, hospital privileges, HMO memberships, and introductions when you speak. If you have not already done so, now is the time to develop this document.

What Is It?

The CV is the medical equivalent of a résumé. It sets out for you and the rest of the world who you are, where you've been, and what you have accomplished along the way. It can trumpet your achievements when modesty might otherwise be expected. It serves as a touchstone for your own self-appraisal. As such, it should be updated on a regular basis throughout your career even when no one else will see it, just to keep you on track and remind you of your goals (and accomplishments).

Unlike the résumé used in the business world, the CV is a recitation of dates, places, and accomplishments. The business résumé generally contains elements such as employment or career goals and objectives, job assignments or performance, and summaries of projects overseen or tasks accomplished. Unlike in the business world, when you use your CV for employment, the job descriptions and your expectations of them are already well defined before you apply. Details of your performance in specific assignments are left to the interview or letters of recommendation, and are not part of the more skeletal CV. This makes the medical résumé simpler to create and maintain but blunts its use as a billboard for you as a candidate. Despite this, there are many ways to create a CV that is an effective tool for your residency application and beyond.

The Effective CV

To be effective, your CV should be neat, clear, well organized, and professional. It should be logically arranged, and inclusive, but spare. It should quickly convey the facts of your accomplishments without excess verbiage or obfuscatory phraseology. It should reflect the chronology of your professional education and experience in an unbroken sequence. Your CV should be visually attractive and uncluttered but not to the extent of gimmickry or unnecessary length. Since your list of accomplishments is still growing at this stage of your career, a CV should be limited to one page if possible. Two pages may be justified in some cases, but not if the content appears stretched or lost in tundral margins of white space.

While the content of the CV is somewhat fixed, the efficacy of the CV can still be enhanced based on your planned use. (Later in your career, you may be in a position or institution that specifies the content and sequence of the CV, but at this point, you have some latitude.) If you are pursuing a field that emphasizes research, any research experience you have had should be highlighted by placing it early and in a prominent position. If you are going to follow a primary care path, your community involvement and commitment to volunteer organizations should come to the fore. If you are pursuing a very competitive position (and you have strong grades), you might include your grade point average when listing your educational institutions, while most of the time this would be omitted. (Your grades from medical school will be shown on the transcript supplied by your dean's office and, therefore, are not generally included in the CV.)

While the CV must be scrupulously factual, the CV is also designed to present you in the best light possible. This is accomplished in both content and form.

Contents and Structure

There are a number of both required and optional elements in the average curriculum vitae (Table 9-1). Some elements are open to interpretation, while others are inflexible. There are entries that are only found in applications at this stage of your career and others that emerge as you mature professionally. We will look at each of these in turn.

Table 9-1 Contents of the "average" CV

```
[Heading]
  Name
  Address
  Biographic / Personal
  Educational
  [Certification]
  [Professional:
    Academic / clinical appointments
    Administrative positions
    Grants obtained]
  Awards/Honors
  Societies/Memberships
  [Community activities]
  [Presentations:
    Oral presentations
    Posters
    Multimedia]
  [Publications:
    Non-peer reviewed
    Abstracts
    Peer reviewed
    Books and chapters]
  {Personal (Hobbies, skills, language)}
  {References}
```

Items shown in italics are unlikely to be part of your CV at this stage of your career. Items in square brackets are optional. Items in curly brackets are generally only included at this stage and are omitted from later versions of your CV.

Heading: If used, this is usually just "Curriculum Vitae." Some advisors think this is superfluous and self-apparent while others think it is business-like and identifies it for what it is. The choice is yours.

Name: This should be your full name, to the extent that you use it everyday or professionally. You may use a middle initial or include your middle name at your discretion. If your name has changed, or it might be the subject of confusion, it should be clarified by a parenthetical entry. The name you use here should match the one you use for you applications and correspondence.

Address: The address you use should be the one where you get your everyday mail. If this will change during the application process (such as with a prolonged out-of-town rotation) you can provide an alternate address with the dates it should be used. If you do not know the -address, you should either provide an update later or have someone trusted screen your mail for important correspondences in your absence. (Another alternative is to include your parents' address as a backup.) The inclusion of a telephone number is a personal decision, but this information is relatively secure and the ability to reach you probably outweighs any privacy concerns. If you have a fax number or e-mail address, consider including them.

Biographic and personal: This section of your CV can be used to adjust the spacing of information on the page. This is because this section is one of the most free form. You may choose to omit much or all of it or to include your birth date and place of birth, marital status, spouse's name, children (with names and birth dates), military service, or social security number. If you include family information, it should be restricted to you and a spouse; do not include your parents. Citizenship is sometimes included in this section. If you are a foreign national, and you choose to include this information, your visa or immigration status should be noted. Some institutions require the inclusion of race or gender for the purposes of the Equal Employment Opportunities Act compliance. At this stage of your career, this is generally not included and is potentially inflammatory. (Indeed, many institutions that once required it from their applicants or employees are moving away from obtaining this information by way of the CV.)

Education: This section is where you list educational institutions you have attended. The list is generally in reverse chronological order (current first) and includes the institution's location (at least the city) and the dates of your attendance. Any degrees or certificates attained should be included. In the case of your medical school, your anticipated degree and date of expected graduation are acceptable. If you performance was stellar, you can choose to include your grade point average. Since this is included in your transcripts, it is optional and should only be added if it was outstanding. The inclusion here of honors gained is a stylistic one since there is a separate section that may be included for that purpose. If you include them here, omit the honors and awards section later. Some advisors favor including your high school while others suggest that the list should only go as far back as your undergraduate school. At this stage of your career, the question is mainly stylistic. If you choose to include it, this will be one of the last times it would be acceptable; remove it before you use your CV for application to a fellowship or postresidency job.

Certification: Later in your career, this is where you will list your medical licensure. At this stage, you should list any special licenses or certifications you do have such as nursing (R.N., L.P.N., etc.), EMT, ACLS, ATLS, or similar. Most students will omit this section.

Professional: As your career evolves, this section will include a listing of your clinical and academic appointments, administrative appointments, and committees on which you serve. If you serve as an officer, this should be noted as part of the entry for that committee or organization. If you participate in task forces, special commissions, or act as a journal reviewer, this section is where you would report those activities. Later in your career, this section is often where you might list any research or other grants and monetary awards obtained. If you have participated in research projects, you can list them here or create a separate heading. Since the research experience most students will have had is likely to be along the lines of employment, rather than supervision or direction of a project, this experience can be listed as work experience if you wish. If you list research experience, list the principal investigator as well.

Awards and honors: If you have received any honors and special recognitions they may be placed in this section, along with the date they were received (if they have not been listed elsewhere). This can include merit-based scholarships, special recognition such as a prize paper, teaching award, competitive fellowship, or the like. In general, this would not include awards received during high school such as NHS or National Merit Scholar. Dean's lists from undergraduate school would be acceptable. You should include a single-sentence description for any honor that is not self-explanatory; sentence fragments are acceptable. The inclusion of this section and its contents are a function of your accomplishments and personal taste. If you have been accorded honors, they should be evident in your CV, but how you choose to highlight them is somewhat flexible. Some students include their scores on certifying examinations ("the Boards") in this section. This, too, is a matter of taste and the scores you got. Unless they are exceptional, this is information that is contained elsewhere or can be provided in other ways. Service as a class officer could be listed here, or under the professional heading.

Societies and memberships: If you have become a member of any regional or national professional organizations, they should be listed under this heading. This might include the student section of the American Medical Student Association (AMSA) or a specialty society, the Student National Medical Society, or others. If you are a member of a professional society related to your undergraduate degree, it can be listed here as well.

Community activities: As your career progresses, you will probably become active as a leader in your community, and this is the place to highlight that involvement. You may have already begun giving back to the community by way of local programs or service projects through your medical school. These illustrate your personal interests, involvement, and initiative. They provide a glimpse into other aspects of you as an individual and help to distinguish you from other applicants. If you had a special role in the project, you can convey it is a descriptive sentence (but no more). Entries in this area are fertile ones for discussion during the interview, so be prepared for possible questions. Many students will include employment experience under this heading, while other will create a separate entry. If you choose to include work experience, you should limit it to significant experience or that which is medically related. It should also be limited to experience during undergraduate and medical school unless it represents the reason for a discontinuity in your educational path. A summer job flipping burgers or watching toddlers may have been critical to your ability to pay for school, but does not contribute to your job qualifications for residency and beyond and can be safely omitted.

Presentations: During residency and beyond, you may have an opportunity to present lectures, research results, or other material in an oral presentation, poster display, or multimedia format. This section chronicles these activities. During your student years, no one expects that you would have had this type of professional experience, but if you have, it should be highlighted. Presentations on rounds or to a small group do not count, but if you were asked to present a grand rounds during one of your rotations, that could be included if you like. Participation as a presenter at a class or school seminar, a poster at a local health fair, or slide show acquainting prospective students with your school would all be worth listing. If you are unsure, check with your advisor for guidance.

Publications: Few students will have publications to their credit at this point in their life. If you do, great. If you don't, it is not a failing, even in the most competitive programs. (If it is, they are not being realistic in their expectations and you may want to reevaluate their desirability.) If you do have publications to your name, they should be listed in chronological order, with the oldest first. The format should be the standard format used by medical journals (or the *Reader's Guide* for non-medical publications). As your lists of published contributions grows, most people separate non-peer reviewed publications, abstracts, peer reviewed , and books and chapters into separate sections with their own heading. As with other aspects of the CV, if you don't have anything to put in, don't include the heading. If you have entries in this section, you may want to move it up in the hierarchy. Some advisors suggest that you highlight your name in any list of references by using boldface type or all capital letters. This is up to you and whatever style seems best based on the overall look of your CV.

Personal: Information about your hobbies, skills, languages spoken, or outside interests is included in your CV only when you are applying for a residency. Once you are in a residency, this information should be deleted. Like community involvement, this area can be used to differentiate you from other candidates. It is also a common point of discussion during the interview process. As a result, don't list a language unless you are fluent—you may get an interviewer who knows the language as well and wants to brush up by carrying out the interview in your native tongue.

References: While entries in this section may show up in your CV later in your career, this is often the only time this information is included. Many students will omit this section even in the CV they use for residency application, preferring instead to provide the information separately. If you use an electronic application system, information about references, along with the associated letters of recommendation, will automatically accompany your application. When you apply for a postresidency job or fellowship, this information is often included in a cover letter, making inclusion in your CV optional even then.

If you have not created a CV for yourself in the past, you might want to start by collecting possible inclusions. This can be done in any form you like, but a sheet of paper or file card for each heading can be useful for recording possible inclusions. This also allows you to reshuffle the sequence you want to use when the time comes to prepare the final version. (If you are a high-tech kind of person, this can be done on a word processor or database program on the computer as well, but it does not require this level of sophistication for just the collection phase.)

If you use the ERAS Student Workstation Software, it provides a CV generator. Based on the information you provide for the Common Application Form, the CV includes information on your educational, professional, and personal history. Data regarding your education, work and research experience, volunteer activities, publications, hobbies, and personal accomplishments can be printed by the residency programs or by you in a "CV report". The format that prints from the Student Workstation is the same format that prints at residency programs. You may choose to use this to summarize your information for you, which you then reformat into your own style of CV. You should create your own paper version even if you use the Student Workstation Software to develop this preliminary version.

While the content of the CV is somewhat standardized, the form that your CV takes can be as individual as you are, within reason. (Some possible layouts are shown in Figures 9-1 through 9-3.) The layout you choose should be clear-cut, readable, and well organized. It can reflect your personal touch and individuality. Some students prefer to place headings along the left side while others want them centered above the pertinent information. Some like horizontal lines to separate sections, others use vertical lines for accents, and others use none at all. (If you use vertical lines, you must use only one or two.) Some students like to include dates on the left, some on the right, and others include them in the information itself. It is all up to you. See what you like. Express yourself and your own style. With your CV, conformity is not required.

As you are considering the look of your CV, give some thought to the sequence you want to use to present the information. The first part is somewhat fixed—you have to give the necessary name, rank, and serial number types of things first so the reader knows who this is all about. After that, you have options. If your strengths lie in honors, research, and publications (you're sure you're not a junior faculty?), put these in early. If you are trying to demonstrate your commitment to your fellow man, move the community and volunteer list up. Lead with your strength—you may have only a limited amount of time to make an impression. The only things that almost always bring up the rear are your hobbies, interests, and references. These are seldom moved above the bottom of the page. These are also the most vulnerable if you should have to make cuts to keep your CV on a single page.

While applications, interviews, and deadlines may seem like a long way off, you should work on your CV early in the process. The process of constructing the CV provides a good opportunity for self-assessment. It can give you the ego boost you need to set your goals higher or the reality check to keep your feet on the ground. You will need time to have your advisor review the preliminary draft for suggestions and to help assess your competitiveness. You will also need to have finished copies ready to give to those you have asked to write letters of recommendation on your behalf. By giving them your CV, you remind them of who you are, and of their promise to write the letter in a timely manner, and you provide substance that can be included in the body of the letter. The result is that you get a better letter, and your strengths may be presented to a reviewer through several different paths.

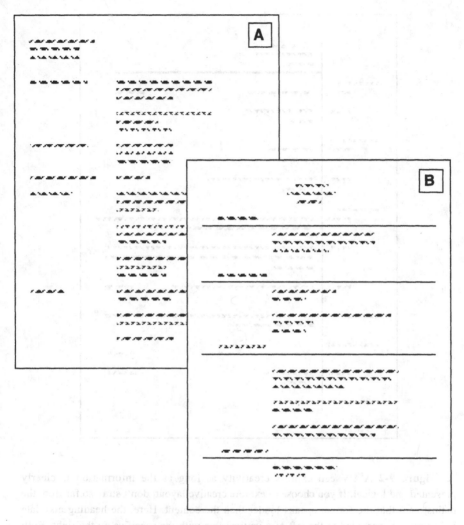

Figure 9-1 A CV can take many different forms. The essential element is neatness and clarity. The use of separators, centering, indentations, and varied margins provides style and visual appeal without resorting to gimmicks or confusing the reader. Example A begins with a name and address in the upper left and uses headings along the left side with a wide indentation of the content to form a visual offset of the material. Example B also begins with a name and address, but this time it has been centered. Content headings are set apart from the content itself by horizontal lines in addition to the use of a wide indententation.

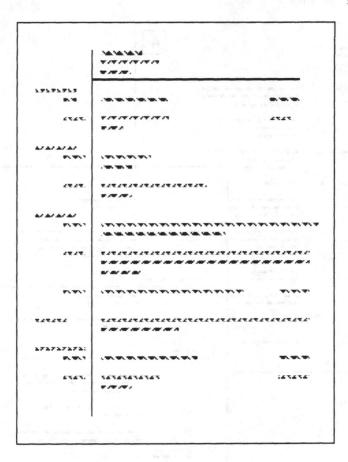

Figure 9-2 A CV can express creativity as long as the information is clearly presented and logical. If you choose to explore creative layout, don't stray so far from the mainstream that the format speaks louder than the content. Here, the heading and date information is provided to the left of a vertical line with the specifics on the right. Both the heading and subheadings have been moved to the left of the vertical separator. Dates have been provided but moved flush to the right-hand margin.

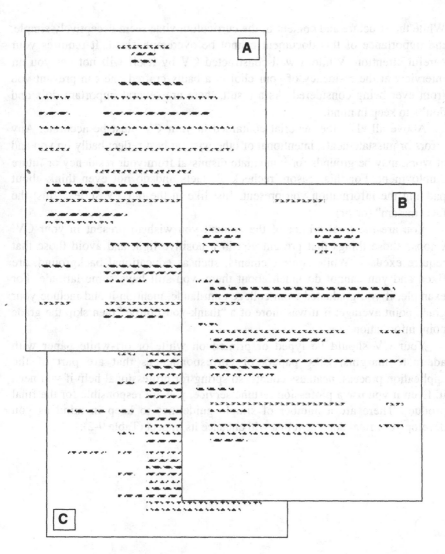

Figure 9-3 These are other common forms the CV may take. The placement of headings, dates, and specifics may be moved around to provide visual appeal. In example A, we once again see a centered name and address, but headings are centered with dates along the left side. The student has chosen to set off the central portion (without date information) by moving the left-hand margin to use the entire width of the page. This can be very effective for calling attention to something like the description of a special award or accomplishment. In B, the student's name acts as the header with two different addresses (mailing and home) flanking the top of the page. Headings are provided with date information aligned with the right margin. Example C places headings, dates, and information in their own visual columns.

Do's and Don'ts

While the structure and content of the curriculum vitae seem deceptively simple, the importance of this document cannot be overemphasized. It requires your careful attention. While a well-constructed CV by itself will not get you an interview at the residency of your choice, a badly crafted one can prevent you from ever being considered. As a result, there are several important do's and don'ts to keep in mind:

Above all else, the material contained in your CV must be accurate. Any errors or misstatements, intentional or otherwise, at best reflect badly on you and at worst may be grounds for immediate dismissal from your residency or future employment. For this reason, recheck all facts and do not even think about padding the information you present. Just like in the old TV series, "Just the facts ma'am" (or sir).

You are the final arbiter of the content you wish to present in your CV. Choose those things that present you in a positive light and avoid those that require excuses. While some elements, such as educational background, are fixed and you cannot do much about them, you still have some latitude. For example, if you graduated from college cum laude, mention it and include your grade point average; if it was more of a "thank-you-Lordy," then skip the grade point information.

Your CV should be typed or printed on white or off-white paper with adequate margins. Like papers or correspondences that are part of the application process, neatness counts, so spring for professional help if you need it. Even it you use a profession résumé service, you are responsible for the final product. There are a number of simple guidelines to keep in mind as you develop your final document that will enhance its impact (Table 9-2).

Table 9-2 Stylistic Guidelines for a Curriculum Vitae

- Your CV must be typed or computer (laser) printed—no exceptions. (Even the typewriter should be your last resort.)
- Use a heavyweight (20–24 pound) bond paper in a neutral color—white or off-white is best. Colored papers can be used, but be careful that you don't leave the impression of gimmickry or artifice. Colored paper is difficult to copy and most programs will have to make extra copies at some point.
- Margins should be generous (1—1.5 inches) unless this results in a few lines flowing onto a second page. (It would be extraordinary to be able to justify more than two pages at this stage of your career, so limit it to two pages; one if possible.)
- Use only one side of the paper if your content flows to a second page.
- Fonts should be 12- to 14- point in size and easily readable. Serif fonts make a good base text with sans serif fonts for headings. Stick to only one or two fonts; any more will just be distracting.
- Limit the use of styles (boldface, italics, small caps) and bullets. What ever you do, <u>don't underline</u>.
- Be consistent with punctuation and capitalization.
- Avoid abbreviations. It is too easy to misinterpret them, and they suggest sloppiness and a lack of care.
- Do not split a section across a page break—rearrange the order of sections or change margins.
- If you use a second page, use a page number at a minimum and strongly consider a header with your name so it can be reunited with the first sheet if it becomes lost.
- Print you final copy on a high-quality laser printer and be sure it photocopies well.

If you are unfamiliar with the styles used in CVs, or English is not your first language, consult a style manual or one of the readily available paperback books on interviews and résumés written for the business world. (If you go this route, be aware of the differences between the business résumé and the medical CV.)

If you have the option, develop your draft copies on a computer so that it can do spelling and grammar checking as you work. This does not prevent the use of a correctly spelled but inappropriate word from getting through, but it helps.

When you think you have finished your CV, have your advisor, a trusted friend, or even your parents go over it for any last-minute suggestions or typos that may have crept in. It is better to have them find the errors than the residency director.

Chapter 10
Effective Personal Statements

Great opportunities engender the greatest challenges. One of the most difficult parts of the application process is the crafting of a personal statement. This free-form test of ingenuity, stamina, and writing skills is the only portion of the application that you have complete control over (sort of). You decide the content, the structure, and the form. It is a personal expression of you, your abilities, interest, and background. It is an opportunity to express your individuality, point out your superiority to other candidates, and pique the interest of the selection committee. It can make or break an application. It will be one of the most difficult pieces of one-page writing you will ever tackle.

Why the Personal Statement?

The personal statement provides a chance to tell the selection committee something special about you. You get to share a glimpse of your interests and abilities, life experiences, and philosophy. You can convey your perspective on life, the reasons for choosing your specialty track, and the special qualifications that make you the person they want. The statement is your surrogate in the first stage of interviews; it speaks for you, arguing your case for an interview and a position in their residency. Like a good movie trailer, it should arouse interest, attract attention, and compel someone to learn more.

Some programs will specify the content or form of the personal statement, but this is becoming uncommon. Most programs leave these decisions in your hands. It is this very lack of direction that many students find the most intimidating; we have all gotten very good at following directions and now there are none. You cannot even fall back on past experience because this composition must address different issues than the one you wrote for your medical school application.

With a little thought, the intent of the personal statement is easy to discern. You want your statement to reflect your maturity, sense of balance, intellect, curiosity, enthusiasm, humor, attitude and drive, background, and motivation. The essay should reflect the source and nature or your commitment to medicine and your field of specialization. Your personal statement may express your expectations from a residency program. You may include your long-term goals, though everyone knows these may be indeterminate or subject to change. Your statement can champion your accomplishments or point out achievements that are not reflected in the drier rhetoric of the curriculum vitae. Your statement should paint a compelling portrait of a winning person, someone who would be engaging to meet and gratifying to work with.

Your personal statement will give those who review your application a sense of how you fit with the specialty and with their program specifically. It should reflect your individuality, flair, and demeanor. Creativity, within bounds, is prized because all personal statements carry the same core purpose and, all too often, content. In your personal essay, you express this creativity through composition, elegance, and ingenuity, whereas in your CV you were limited to structural elements and appearance to set you apart. Your composition should demonstrate your clarity of thought and linguistic ability. These varied demands are constrained by the context of a single page of printed text—an intimidating assignment.

The role of the personal statement as your advocate is crucial in the application process. A well-done statement can overcome an otherwise lackluster portfolio; a statement thrown together without care can scuttle the chances of the class valedictorian. The process of fashioning a masterful personal essay must be deliberate and allotted sufficient time to result in a product worthy to be your proxy.

The Painful Process

Several steps are involved in producing an engaging personal statement. First you must decide your objectives for the piece, next the content that will move toward those goals, and lastly the artfulness of language that will express and tie together your ideas. None of these steps is easy and each must be revisited repeatedly over time. This charge demands focus and discipline, a timetable, and trusted friends. It will require hubris and bravado to recount your strengths, and brutal honesty in your revisions. It will cause great angst.

Many students find the most difficult part of the task is deciding where to start. If you set out with a blank page and no clear direction, you will almost certainly founder, unable to place even the first word on the page. A better beginning is to set yourself an assignment with specific goals. What are the ideas you want to convey, the attributes you want to highlight, or the events you want noticed?

The most common topics covered in personal statements are limited to a surprisingly small number (Table 10-1). Most students will choose to cover only a few of these options. Do not feel confined to these areas; let your creativity show. You should pick subject matter that is the most comfortable for you. Pick topics where you shine, are unique, or have something special to say. Look at those that can be woven together to form a theme or thread that draws the reader in, a unified whole that leaves them wanting to learn more. Will you set your narrative in the past (growing up), the present (me today), or the future (where I want to be)? Will you choose an event or location as a setting or example of some point? These decisions will help to give a better picture of where to begin. Some examples to give you ideas of how these elements work are included at the end of this chapter.

Table 10-1 Common Themes in Personal Statements

- Who am I?
- Where have I come from?
- What have I accomplished?
- Why have I chosen this field?
- What are my career plans or goals?
- What can I contribute?

By no means should you feel constrained to themes common to most personal essays. They are the easiest to imagine and use as a starting point, but are not required. There is no limit to the material that might be considered even if you stay with the well-tested themes most often used:

Who am I? This approach allows you to present a special look at you, the person. What are your strength and weaknesses? How would others describe you? What are your outside interests? Ask yourself, Do I have an area of special knowledge, expertise, or experience, such as hobbies, avocations, second careers, special course work, or the like? These add depth to you as a person and candidate. This approach allows you to show off unusual skills or experiences. Have you done something special or traveled somewhere unusual, and how has that changed you, made you a better person, doctor, or candidate? Material of this type is the easiest to come by but potentially the weakest of that in the six main types. If done extraordinarily well, some of the most intriguing statements can still come from this material. (I remember one that began, "I am writing this while paddling down a river in Guatemala" and another that began with the student walking along the streets of Disneyland.)

Where have I come from? This autobiographical approach is customarily filled with stories of parents, siblings, and life-changing events. While these are interesting, if you go this route be sure that there is a clear message or reason for the recounting. How did these factors influence your abilities, character, demeanor, or decision to pursue medicine or a particular specialty? If you choose this route, avoid trite scenarios or emotional tumult, which too easily become melodramatic, inflated in significance, or difficult to believe. (Do you really think a residency director is going to believe that your choice of specialty was caused by an alien encounter? Do you really want them to?) Make sure that any story you relate has a beginning, middle, and end and is clearly relevant to your point.

What have I accomplished? This approach allows you to enumerate those special things that you have accomplished or achieved that are not reflected elsewhere in your application. Do not recapitulate your CV—you just spent time making sure it could stand on its own, now let it. This might include the recognition of your work with a volunteer organization (most nails hammered for Habitat for Humanity, a new logo for a homeless shelter), or an unusual life experience (walking the Appalachian Trail, finding a new fossil). If you recount this kind of story, it should have a clear-cut end (accomplishment of a goal) and have some bearing on you as a residency candidate. Keep the accomplishment in perspective. Why was it special? How did you grow from the experience? How will it make you a better doctor or resident? The accomplishment you recount may be the triumph over an obstacle, hardship, or handicap. You can use this form to explain a problem in your past or control damage. (No, a letter from your parole officer is not as strong as a letter of recommendation from a mentor or service chief.) If you go this route, don't dwell on the negative. The last impression you want to leave is a negative or depressing one.

Why have I chosen this field? Like the "who am I" area of discussion, this is an easy out, but filled with potential traps and dangers. We all know the attributes of each field of medicine, their rewards and special joys. Everyone recognizes the satisfaction of constructing something with your hands (surgery), solving a riddle (internal medicine), helping a child (pediatrics), or being present at the miracle of birth (obstetrics, and sometimes emergency medicine). The problem is that when you put these things in your personal statement, you are preaching to the choir. The folks that read your statement have been there and done that, and probably appreciate these things even more than you do. Consequently, you are unlikely to be sufficiently eloquent to impress, and you can use the space for better things. If you really can't come up with anything else, then use this but make it relevant to you, your background and skills, and your candidacy for residency. Never, ever, mention monetary or lifestyle issues as the reason for your choice.

What are my career plans or goals? This line of discussion is fraught with risk. It is all too easy to say that you would like "a rural clinical practice with the possibility of involvement in teaching and research." Vague generalities are more damaging than helpful. If you have a strong set of career plans, go ahead and point them out, but put them in perspective. Tell the reader how these fit with your skills, personality, ability, or specialty choice. A clear vision of yourself and your future can be a very positive attribute, though no residency director expects it at this stage of your professional life.

What can I contribute? These points are often folded in with your accomplishments, skills, or special attributes cataloged in other ways. These may be qualifications that are not documented by specific accomplishments or ones that stem from your upbringing. Why are you a better candidate than the others who will cross the selection committee's desk in the next few weeks? Tell the readers why their residency needs you. Don't be pompous, condescending, or outlandish. Do state your capabilities with pride (and supporting examples or data). You can express self-confidence and self-worth without being arrogant. Don't forget that they are looking for a resident, not a fellow, researcher, or section chief, so stay focused on the job you are seeking.

Once you have decided on a basic strategy for your personal statement, begin writing. Rough out your statement and then let it sit for a few days or a week or even two. After this gestation period, evaluate what you have written. When you go back to your statement you will be amazed at what you said and how badly it was written. [If you are not, there are two possibilities: (1) you do not understand the process, or (2) you need to consider employment as a dean.] Go through your work. Cut unnecessary words or paragraphs, rewrite sections that do not make sense, and rethink the flow of ideas. Set this version aside for a while and then repeat the process for as many times as it takes to get something that seems serviceable. This is your *first* draft.

Once the first draft of your personal statement is ready, share it with your advisor. (You can also use a trusted friend or spouse, though this can threaten the relationship unless it is strong and your ego is prepared.) Ask your advisor to go over the statement, searching for areas where the thoughts, flow, or grammar can be strengthened. (Remember that the responsibility for the initial grammar checking is yours—you only want your advisor to give you suggestions for better sentence structures, more lively language, or improved word usage.) Ask him or her to comment on the ability of the composition to draw in the reader, generate interest, improve your desirability, or explain away problems. Take the suggestions you receive and look at your work for ways to address the concerns raised. Can you incorporate some or all of the suggestions without violating your own sense of style, rhythm, or modesty?

Once you make the necessary changes to your first draft, repeat the evaluation process by returning to your advisor with this version. When you are both happy with your work, again put the piece aside. Revisit it for the last time just before you are ready to file it with your applications and give it to those who will write letters of recommendation. If it is ready, print your statement (or have it printed) on a high-quality bond paper using a laser printer. (If you have used an unusual paper for printing your CV, use the same paper for your personal statement.) Make lots or original copies; you don't want anyone receiving something that appears to be a photocopy.

One or Many?

The question of making more than one form of the personal statement is becoming easier with the advent of electronic applications, which send one personal statement to all of the programs to which you apply. If you are applying using a paper application, you might consider using personal statements that are customized for each program. This can be as simple as a version targeted toward university programs and another with more of a community program viewpoint. Word processing and mail merging can push this concept to the extreme of personal statements made to order for each program.

From a practical standpoint, you neither have the time nor should take it to write completely different personal statements. This task is tough enough that your efforts should be undivided in the quest of one excellent statement rather than several mediocre ones. What can be done is to modify one or two sentences or a paragraph so that they reflect slightly different aspects of you or your goals. If you are applying to a university or research-oriented program, you can emphasize past experiences or abilities that are relevant. If you are applying to a community program, statements that reflect your commitment to service or community involvement can be showcased.

The simplest method for customization is to insert the name of the institution into a statement such as: "The reputation of [NAME OF PROGRAM] for its excellence in teaching, research, and clinical experience makes your program a logical choice for someone like myself." This can be manually inserted just befor you print each copy of the statement or can be automated with the use of a mail merge and a list of programs. This technique is the easiest of the options.

Is it worth doing? The reality is that, while it is a nicety, a custom-tailored personal statement is not as much of an asset as is an innovative, imaginative, or memorable one. If you are applying by a paper application and a sentence that lends itself to modification is a logical part, go ahead. Otherwise, don't force the issue, go with one good statement.

Do's and Don'ts

Many secrets can help make or break a personal statement. Most of these suggestions are simple common sense; others are less obvious. All are easy to use in any style of personal statement.

Things to Do

- **Think about who will read your statement.** Like any good presentation, you need to know your audience. Think about what you would be looking for if you were reading this as a part of the selection committee. What attributes would set you apart or make you a good resident in your chosen field? If you are unsure, ask your advisor about what he or she looks for when reading student statements. Structure your essay with this in mind.

- **Grab the reader's attention.** The first few sentences of your essay will be what "sells" the rest. While most of the readers of your personal statement do not have a choice (it is part of being on the committee), you don't want them bored or skipping to the end. For this reason, you will want a "grabber." This can be an anecdote or an unusual turn of phrase or observation. Use action verbs and short sentences to convey an active pace. Your statement does not have to begin with an introductory paragraph; you can jump directly into the substance.

- **Keep the reader's attention.** Use a lively writing style with varied sentence structure and length. Move your story in a logical manner from point to point so that the reader never becomes sidetracked.

- **Clarity sells.** Be clear in your writing. Avoid the passive voice. Use the correct words or phrases to carry your message. Use a thesaurus liberally to ensure variety and the best word for the task. Make every sentence count—you only have one page.

- **Be specific in your statements and points:** Generalities only muddy the water. Be concrete.

- **Be consistent in you tone and content.** Don't portray yourself as meteoric if your transcript say you are just another rock. Don't tell the reader you want to find a cure for cancer and then turn around and say you want a rural practice in an underserved area.

- **Preempt concerns.** If there are significant questions that might be raised about your candidacy, address them up front and in a forthright manner. These might include medicine as a second career, your age, or family concerns. Turn these issues into positives: Your age gives you maturity, your youth brings stamina, a family provides stability, and so forth. Check with your advisor to be sure there really is a concern before you raise the issue.

- **Give the reader something to remember.** Just like a memorable opening, you will want a strong finish. Leave the reader with something positive to remember about you.

- **Edit and proofread carefully.** If possible, compose your essay on a computer word processor with the ability to check spelling and grammar. Computer spelling checkers can only tell you if the collection of letters you have typed is in a list (dictionary) of acceptable words. They can't tell if you typed in the name of a type of Norwegian fjord when you meant to use a preposition. The onus falls to you to read and reread your work for this type of error. Grammar checking programs are not as sophisticated, but will seldom create major problems, so use their evaluations as advisory. Use friends who were English majors in a past life or pay a professional editor to make a final pass just to be sure.

- **Neatness counts.** Just like your CV, neatness counts. Lay out your statement with ample margins—generally 1 to 1.5 inches on the sides and a minimum of 1 inch on the bottom. Choose an easy to read font (Table 10-2) and use it consistently throughout your paper. Unlike the CV where more than one font may be desirable to set apart various sections, changing fonts here will be distracting. Serif fonts are often easier to read than are sans serif types. The choice is personal and will depend on the font size you choose. What ever you settle on, be sure it is easily readable by the older members of the selection committee.

Table 10-2 Commonly Used Fonts

Serif Fonts	San Serif Fonts
Times Roman (what this book is set in)	Arial
Bookman	**Charcoal**
Century Schoolbook	Geneva
Courier	Helvetica

- **Identify your work.** If your statement will be separate from your application (such as with a paper application), put your name and NRMP student number at the top or bottom of your essay. After all this work, you would hate to have your personal statement filed with some other student's application.

Things to Avoid

- **Avoid self-serving statements.** Let statements speak for you without having to resort to an excessive use of the first person singular ("I" for those of you entering the surgical specialties).
- **Don't use gimmicks.** While the structure of your statement is up to you, the readers of your statement will generally be a conservative group. Something done just for effect (writing your entire statement as a bawdy limerick) is likely to make the committee question your

stability rather than note your creativity. You can still convey enthusiasm, inventiveness, wit, and intellect in a more traditional structure.

- **Avoid clichés like the plague.** Trite and overused phrases, like the one I just used, turn off the reader and suggest laziness on your part—not the impression you want to leave. There are better ways to express yourself.
- **Don't abbreviate.** Except in telling an anecdote, contractions and abbreviations should not be used. There are few better ways to turn off a selection committee than to use an abbreviation or slang term for the field of study you are considering.
- **Avoid emotional entanglements.** Emotions, whether it is a heart-rending story or expressions of overarching altruism, can easily backfire. They are almost never needed and carry too high a risk of diverting your message.
- **Don't include inflammatory statements.** Statements about the advantages or shortcomings of a geographic area, particular program, or field of study risk alienating part or all of your audience. Talking about the glories of the Midwest will turn off the folks from other regions. Talking badly about another program or field of medicine suggests you are shallow and petty. Even in the context of an interview, these are dangerous positions to take.
- **Don't give away the store.** While you can use the personal statement to help explain a problem in your past, don't call attention to problems if they are not significant. Having honors in only one-third of your courses would not be seen as problem until you point it out. Unless your advisor suggests that damage control is in order, don't leave the selection committee with a negative impression. The last thing you need is to be seen as someone who whines and makes excuses.
- **Avoid gratuitous anecdotes and humor.** Any personal story you choose to include must have a clear message related to your central point. It must reflect intelligence and insight, not just your presence at the event. What (specifically) did you learn? What message did it send? Why was it important? While self-effacing humor can be effective when used sparingly, it is risky and best avoided.
- **Don't get in over your head.** Don't make statements that reflect an unrealistic appraisal of your abilities or the demands of the job ahead. Telling a selection committee that you will simultaneously be the best resident they have, run a day care center, and compose an opera in their honor will not be believed. You don't want to make statements that you cannot defend during an interview or deliver on during the years of residency.
- **Avoid the syrup.** Don't pour it on too thick. A heavy-handed recounting of your abilities or qualifications will come off as condescending. Give the committee a little credit—lead them gently.

Examples

Got some basic ideas? Here are some excerpts from actual personal statements submitted by students over the past couple of years. (Yes, they are all now residents.) Each illustrates a particular technique or point. No single personal statement can or should include all of the elements demonstrated here. Some may give you ideas that fit your style, while others that are excellent in their own context will seem stilted, stiff, or contrived in your statement.

A Great Opening

In their opening paragraphs, our first examples use two different techniques to draw you in and make you want to know more about the candidate.

> I had gone to bed late that evening after attempting to study just a few more pages of one of those big medical books. My eyelids heavy, I had crawled into bed and sleep had come quickly and easily. Then I began to have an annoying dream about a phone that was ringing incessantly. Wait! That was no dream. Suddenly, I was wide awake to the voice of the Family Practice doctor with whom I was working, saying (at 3:30 A.M., I noted), "You're needed at the hospital—we've got an emergency C-section coming in by squad from a town 40 miles away." Immediately I rushed to the small 20-bed hospital, where our patient arrived minutes later. Before I knew it, I found myself in the assistant's position, suction in hand, set for my first delivery. Gush!! I was caught off guard by this unexpected barrage of fluid as well as the miraculous appearance of an 8-lb. 3-oz baby boy.

Yes, I'm hooked. In this example, while a bit melodramatic, there is energy, a change of pace and rhythm, an urgency and excitement. While anyone who delivers babies has "been there, done that," the paragraph piques an interest in how this affected this candidate, what lessons were learned, and how this influenced the student's career decisions.

> In 1989, I was working twelve hours per day as a courier in our city. One particularly busy afternoon I had to make a pickup in downtown and I was running a few minutes late. I hurriedly parked my car in one of the underground garages and ran up to street level where rush hour traffic was congested and thick. I was obsessively thinking about how best to get into and out of the office building. My impatience with the stoplights and traffic was mounting as I stepped off the sidewalk and into the street. I had not noticed the gigantic red bus churning down the street several yards in front of me.

In this example, just like in a good suspense movie, I <u>have</u> to know what happens next. O.K., here are his next three paragraphs:

> But a longhaired gentleman standing next to me had noticed. He calmly grabbed my shirt collar and gave a solid tug. I nearly fell onto my backside. My immediate reaction was one of anger, until I felt the hot swirl of bus exhaust coiling around my body and realized that I had come within inches of being smashed against the pavement by several tons of rush hour bus.
>
> "Slow down, man," was all he said.
>
> He turned and slowly walked away as I tried to collect my wits amidst the rush of adrenaline and pedestrians. Rudely confronted with my own mortality, I vowed to "slow down" and proceed with gratitude.

Even though I now know the outcome of the close encounter, I still want to know more about this student. In the rest of his statement he tells us how his life, medical school, and the death of his father all shaped who he is, where he is going, and what he wants to accomplish with his life. He brings it full circle with his simple closing statement:

> I await that opportunity, and in the meantime, I will proceed with gratitude.

This is someone you want to interview.

Bringing Closure

The technique of bringing closure, the way a good short story does, can be accomplished in many ways. In our next example, the student opened her statement by saying that she was proud to say that her parents, and their values, have been guiding forces in her life. This is even truer after their deaths, which occurred while she was in medical school. She uses the final paragraph to fold those attributes into her value as a candidate and future resident.

> Since these profound losses, I have vowed to implement the ethics my parents instilled in me. The field I have chosen will allow me to do so with passion and drive. I will continue to fight for the health and safety of my patients. I will practice disease prevention and health maintenance. My manual skills as a violinist will be revealed through surgical precision. I will attempt to discover new relationships to disease through clinical research. I will strive to enhance my community through public health programs and clinics. I will make it my life's work to make a difference in my patients' lives, just as my parents have made a difference in my life.

Yes, there is the problem that this women wants to be everything for everybody—a clinician, teacher, scientist—but you get the sense she just might do it.

The personal glimpse can be effective, but it often takes up space you may not want to commit. If you still like this approach, one solution is to be sure your message and point of the story is evident early in the telling, as in our next example:

> "I'll take him!" I exclaimed proudly as a young child and picked up the smallest, skinniest, most feeble kitten in the bunch. My parents allowed me to choose the family pet, for the first time. After the first cat died, I chose others, and all were the runts of the litter. I would take them home, feed them, and love them. Soon they would grow to be the largest, sleekest, and prettiest cats in the neighborhood. One kitten had to be fed around the clock with an eyedropper. Tired as I was, I always made sure that my alarm was set to wake me for his feedings. These early memories, the first indication that I was heading toward a life of service to others, taught me about the responsibility that is needed when taking care of another life. I experienced the joy in giving of one's self expecting nothing in return, yet gaining a priceless gift of love and self-satisfaction.

Family Values

Family values are a common theme of personal statements. They are easier to write because you no longer have to write in the first person. Most of us are raised to at least pretend humility, so statements about out own attributes are uncomfortable. By talking about someone else, our parents or family, we get around this problem while still hinting at our own traits by extension. The opening sentence by this next young woman lets you know that she can hold her own.

> Growing up on a ranch in rural South Dakota with five brothers taught me how to be a team player at an early age. My mother and father, who have deep faith, a tremendous work ethic, and a strong commitment to community and family, instilled in me qualities that will make me a good physician. My father, a rancher/carpenter and a pillar in the local church, is a man of integrity. He modeled the sacrifices that must be made to operate a ranch successfully and to live each day with a clear conscience. My mother is the one who sparked my interest in medicine. She loves caring for people and has a very inquisitive mind.

While I am concerned about this woman's architectural father (is he really a pillar?), we get the sense that we are dealing with a down-to-earth, hard-working future resident with integrity and intellect. I know what I am getting with this person, straight up and no games—just get the work done.

Not every candidate has had a Midwestern, apple pie, American flag kind of family that they can be proud of. Many students come from different forms of families: families in conflict, personal hardships, and the kinds of traumas most of us hope to avoid. The decision to recount this type of life experience is difficult. On the one hand, it can illustrate your tenacity and ability to survive; on the other, you can come off as seeking pity. Here is an example of an opening paragraph that presents a family stress in a way that draws you into the narrative without being maudlin.

> One of the remarkable things I have noticed about many doctors is that they have had a personal experience or family history of illness, which became the motivation to initiate their career, or to select a specialty. My case has not been an exception. In 1981, my youngest sister was diagnosed with diabetes mellitus. I was ten and she was seven years old. We stopped "playing doctor" to play real life. Each member of the family assumed new responsibilities for her care. I clearly remember waiting for the change of color of the reactive Clinitest, the maximum technology at the time to evaluate the glucosuria; but I remember even more my hand shaking when I took her arm to inject her insulin doses.

This young woman goes on to tell us of her high school graduation as valedictorian and her path to becoming a residency candidate. We get a glimpse into how this affected her life, but with no apologies, tears, or appeal for sympathy. Over the years, I have read statements that talk of family abuse, alcoholism in one or both parents, personal divorces, broken homes, and tragic losses. Some have been uncomfortable to read—like suddenly finding yourself in the middle of a therapy session without being invited. Some have been presented artfully enough that you did not get the feeling of a daytime soap opera. The best suggestion for those who come from a troubled background is to spend time discussing the options with your advisor. You cannot and should not hide who you are or where you came from, but sometimes you need not flaunt it either.

If you don't want to use your family to suggest your attributes, how do you point them out to the selection committee? Often the best way is to just list them:

> I believe that my knowledge, clinical skills, communication, and technical ability will make me a great physician. Additionally, my empathy, open-mindedness, willingness to advocate for women, commitment, and enthusiasm will make me an excellent doctor. Finally, I believe it is my friendliness, ability to get along with others, love of teaching, and learning from others that will make me the kind of resident you will want. I will bring forth my motivation, willingness to learn, and my undeniable dedication, and will work to earn the confidence and respect of your program.

Any questions? This young woman lays it out for all to see. You don't have to worry about how she got these attributes, just what she will do with them. This is a strong statement that not every student can, or would, make, but this student is comfortable laying it on the line. The statement is a bit dry and it could just as easily have been written as a template by a resume writer and posted on the Internet. It makes assertions about the candidate, but they lack personality. This impersonality, while factual, is not as compelling as some of the other statements we have seen.

Making Choices

Many personal statements will include something about why the applicant chose their particular field of medicine. This can work well, but avoid "preaching to the choir." As we have said above, the selection committee members are all in your chosen field and probably have the same (or a better) vision of the field. Here is one woman's statement that successfully skirts the trite aspects of her choice while still conveying the elements involved in her decision:

> I am attracted to this field because it encompasses continuity of care and exciting technology, broadening its scope beyond primary care medicine. The rotations I enjoyed the most were those that allowed me to be personally involved in procedures. This was most evident during my surgical rotation when I was able to step beyond theory and actively treat a patient, perhaps changing the course of a patient's disease. I was awed by the precision and composure displayed by the surgeon while performing a procedure. Yet, even more fulfilling was seeing the immediate impact the surgery made upon the patient's quality of life.

We learn about the aspects of surgical care that this candidate enjoys but it could be more compelling, involving, or personal. Yes, these are the personal reasons for the student's choice, but we are outsiders, not drawn into the prose the way we were with some of the other statements. If we had had details of the case, the type of surgery involved, or the things the student did when "personally involved," we would have a different feel for this person.

If you feel that you have to make the obvious statements, make them in a less obvious way. This student puts a different spin on surgical anatomy:

> ... The human body can be viewed as a living creation of art, elegantly depicting the intricate synchrony of form and function. In no other field can this be demonstrated more vividly than in our area of medicine.

Some students are able to combine several approaches. Our next example combines the exposition of family values with the problem of making choices in a novel and interesting way.

> ...They all had different plans for my future. My sister Joanne, a veterinarian, thought I would be a surgeon. My biggest fan when I was a high school quarterback and college athlete, she feels I am skillful with my hands and possess the ability to assess, identify, and evaluate problems quickly. My sister Mary, a critical care nurse, suggested that I should be an Emergency Room physician. She describes me as self-confident, caring, and strong willed, qualities that enable me to handle any situation effectively. My mother feels Family Practice or Internal Medicine is my true calling because my kind heart, dedication, and warm personality are best suited to primary care.

This paragraph gives us a lot of information in a very few words. We know about the nature of the student's family, and the attributes he brings to the residency without the dryness that a simple list would have carried. He has let others be the ones to list his strengths on his behalf. We also know something about the student's high school activities and outside interests. Not bad for just six sentences.

Telling a selection committee what you are looking for in a residency can help to get you a good fit. An example that uses this approach to give a sense of where the candidate wants to go is our next excerpt.

> I am interested in a strong didactic program that included challenges and opportunities for both the residents and students, while simultaneously providing the highest quality of care possible for the patients. Presently my plan is to continue my training in a busy and diverse program that has exposure to all subspecialties, as my mind is still open to the further possibilities within the field. I hope that I will be able to utilize my strengths while being challenged academically, and given the privilege to learn more from others.

Yes, we do have another case of everything for everybody, but we know that the student wants a program that will allow flexibility in his future career paths by being both academic and clinically oriented. This combination does exist in most specialties, making this an achievable mix. As a selection committee member, I can now try to decide if I can provide the kind of training the student seeks.

In the Spotlight

As we have noted earlier in this chapter, the personal statement can be used to highlight for the selection committee some accomplishment or achievement. Here is an example:

> Throughout medical school, I have felt that balance in life is essential. During my first year, I joined an organization that emphasizes academic excellence balanced with a more traditional college experience. Our group is committed to philanthropy, scholastics, and a loving and supportive sisterhood. I held several different offices in the group, including president and ritualist. My involvement has enabled me to develop leadership and organizational skills. In addition, I have been fortunate to take an active role in the student sections of the American Medical Association. I had the privilege of attending the 1994 annual meeting in Chicago. Actively participating in this organization has reminded me of the benefits, both personally and professionally, of being a member of a medical society. In addition to these medical school activities, I enjoy spending time walking, jogging, and weight training. All of these activities keep the balance I need to be the best physician possible.

This woman's statement makes sure we know about her accomplishments, but also keeps them in perspective; this is someone who has outside interests, but can maintain an equilibrium with the main task at hand. She is still a student. Her activities in her sorority have been only a part of her medical school experience, but they are a part that she has done well.

Balance can be a strong indicator of stability and insight. In this next excerpt, we get a clear image of responsibility and learn about the student's family at the same time:

> The experiences during my medical education have been diverse. I feel these experiences will assist me in my development as a successful resident and physician. While always striving for academic excellence, I have sought to involve myself with my family, student government, work, and church. My wife, Heidi, and two little girls, Kennedy and Cassidy, are the greatest sources of joy in my life. They have helped me meet the rigors and stresses of medical school, and I know they will continue to be a strength to me in the years ahead.

This student acknowledges that he has a ways to go, both in time and in training, but stresses his diversity of experience and skill. He does this while staying grounded to the constancy of a supportive family. As a selection committee member, he has even addressed any concerns I might have about the possibility of burnout or distraction, since he has already proven his ability to focus on many pursuits at the same time.

The Literary Approach

Sometimes a quote can set the tone of your statement, or may be used to set apart ideas for which you hold strong feelings. If you go this route, the quote should be relevant and of sufficient weight as to be more than name dropping. While this next example could be criticized as preachy or pedagogical, it does allow the student to make a point about both her beliefs and accomplishments while demonstrating a broader education and reading beyond topics in medicine.

> Prudence B. Saur, M.D. wrote in 1887, "The time has arrived when a more diffusive knowledge of the laws of health will be appreciated by the women of our land." More than 100 years later, that observation could not apply more to the women of the 1990s. For instance, I have had the opportunity to use my knowledge to educate other women. On several occasions at a shelter for battered women, I provided lay education on various health topics such as breast self-examination and hypertension. These sessions took place on Saturday mornings and sometimes there were only two or three women present but they listened intently, and despite their current difficult situations they soaked up the information with a fervor not expressed by many. I felt if I reached even one woman it was worthwhile. Additionally, I lectured to college-aged women at a local community college regarding sexually transmitted disease, and to pregnant teenagers at an area high school about proper nutrition during pregnancy. Through these interactive sessions I realized how important a little understanding and personal attention can be to a frightened or confused young women. All these experiences have given me insight into what positive impact my education can have on the lives of others.

The quote provides a nice lead into an exposition of the student's community involvement that might not come through in a simple entry on her curriculum vitae.

As you can see, no two personal statements are alike. That is a good thing, not only because it allows you to be creative, but, speaking for those who have to read these statements, it means a much more interesting task. Now that you have some ideas, start writing.

Chapter 11
Recommendations

All residency applications require letters of recommendation from mentors and others able to judge, and speak to your character, ability, and desirability as a resident. Like your own personal statement, these letters should point out your strengths, providing a strong endorsement of your candidacy. Unlike your personal statement, these letters are designed to be objective and, in most cases, confidential appraisals from those who know you and your work. That does not mean that they are totally out of your control. The selection of who you want to perform this job, and your charge to them, will influence the quality of the letters you get.

Who to Pick?

Getting top-notch letters of recommendation begins with selecting the best letter writers. Some programs will specifically ask for a letter of recommendation from the department chairman at your place of training. With this exception, the choice of evaluators is yours.

You will want to select as evaluators faculty members who have worked closely with you during a rotation or elective. Pick those with whom you had a good rapport, and for whom you performed at your best. Pick those who expressed an interest in writing a letter or were the best teachers. (Good teachers are committed to students and know the value of a good letter.) A little time spent at this stage will result in significantly better letters. Some general guidelines are as follows:

- Get the right people. The letters of recommendation should not come from former employers, family members, clergy, politicians, patients, or residents you have worked with. Unless you are entering a field with a heavy basic science component, letters should not come from your basic science teachers. For all practical purposes, your advocates must come from the clinical faculty in your chosen field. If you have possible champions in a related field, you can consider them, but they will not carry the same weight as an endorser from your specialty.

- Be choosy. Pick only faculty you believe will give you a favorable recommendation. This seems self-evident, but it is critical. Everyone who reads a letter of recommendation knows that the letter writer was hand-selected to put you in the best light. Someone who writes a formula letter or a letter of faint praise can doom you without your even knowing it has happened. This may arise innocently when the letter writer is just too busy to take the time, or if he or she is too inexperienced to know the importance of the task. Be sure every one of your authors will give you a glowing recommendation. If you are not sure, ask. If there is any reason you are still not sure, use someone else.

- Ask early. As you are moving through your clinical rotations, ask potential letter writers if they would be willing to write letters when the time comes. By asking early you "reserve a space" for later and can get a sense of who might do as an endorser. If you have asked early, when you come back to them later in the year they will remember the commitment. If you decide not to use them after all, they will not be hurt (and may not even remember the request).

- Ask often. Although you will only need three or four letters to accompany your application, you should ask up to twice as many people if they would be willing to perform this service. This allows you to spread the work load and to customize the destination of the letters to get maximum benefit.

- Use connections. Select your letter writers with an eye to the programs you are considering. If your letter writer is familiar with (and to) the program you are seeking, the letter will be more personal and carry more weight. Take advantage of the natural tendency to generate a more personal letter when you know the recipient. Letters written from one friend or professional acquaintance to another will always garner more attention. Even with the electronic residency application, you will have the option to decide to which programs each letter is sent. Use this option creatively.

- Go for the top. Pick the most senior faculty members who meet your other requirements. While you may have bonded with the second-year residents during your junior rotation, they are not the best persons to ask for a letter of recommendation. They would certainly have the knowledge of you required and would write a good letter, but they lack the name recognition needed to be powerful spokespersons. Just as in advertising, you believe the endorsement of a star or celebrity over that of the man on the street, even though the latter's opinion may be more germane and considered. Use faculty with "star power," if they can otherwise write a good letter.

- Get experience. Choose faculty who write letters every year. Pick faculty from the selection committee of your own school. These folks know what to put in a letter, what phrases carry weight, and how to say things succinctly.

- Use your advisor. Use your advisor to help pick the best candidates. Use your advisor as a letter writer as well. If you have been getting the most out of your advisor, he or she should know you well by now.

If you are applying to a program that requires a chairman's letter, you will need to do some additional steps. Like letters from other faculty members, you will need to supply the chairman with adequate information upon which to base the letter. Unlike the letter writers you get to choose, your chairman may not know you from the other students who rotate through the department. If your school uses more than one site, you may not even have had your junior rotation in the same institution. To overcome this, you will need to plan several appointments with the chairman to become acquainted. Chairmen tend to be busy with tasks that keep them out of the office (or even out of town). Consequently, you will have to plan so that these visits are unhurried and occur well in advance of the date that you need your letters.

What to Ask Them For?

Most of the faculty you ask for a letter of recommendation will know what is required, but that is not enough. If you only mention your request when passing in the hall and provide a secretary with a list of names and addresses, you are likely to get a bland letter that looks like the product of a mail merge. Faint praise, at best. To get the best letters you need to help your letter writers with substance and specifics.

Start by being sure the authors know you as a person. Make an appointment to talk. Tell them about your plans, aspirations, attributes, and skills. Make them aware of things in your past that should be highlighted and those best avoided. Let them know about your background and upbringing. Tell them about the things that are not in the transcript or your CV. Give them the individual glimpses required to write a letter that is interesting and personal.

Suggest specifics to your letter writers. These faculty are busy and are generally grateful for any direction you give them. Discuss the areas or specific topics that you would like them to cover. Your own strengths and experiences may drive these areas or they may be driven by the styles of the residency you are seeking. If you are pursuing a program that prizes manual skills, then ask your letter writers to focus on these abilities. If you are going into a field that stresses intellectual prowess, ask them to note your board scores, research projects, or publications. If you are going into an area that stresses people-to-people skills, ask them to recount that episode with the kitten and the burning building. Little hints can go a long way to making your letter of recommendation something that promotes you as a residency candidate. Some students provide this nudge with a follow-up letter confirming and formalizing the request (Figure 11-1). This is an excellent idea for many reasons and is strongly encouraged.

August 4, 2000

Dr. Alfred Nobel
Department of Medical Specialty
Old Pooh-Pooh University
Oceanview, IL, 61820

Dear Dr. Nobel:

   Thank you for agreeing to write letters of recommendation on my behalf to your friends at the programs in Stockholm. I hope that you will mention my experience as a research assistant in your laboratory and my extensive work with the poor in Third-World countries. The selection committee might also like to know about my hobby as a formula-one racecar mechanic. To assist you with your writing, I have enclosed a copy of my transcript, personal statement, current CV, and an endorsement from two U.S. Senators.

   So that I can submit my applications in a timely way, I will need these letters by the end of the month. I have supplied your office staff with the names, titles, and mailing addresses of everyone involved.

   Thank you again for your assistance.

Sincerely yours,

Stellar Student

Figure 11-1 A simple note can summarize the content of your meeting with a letter writer and serve as a gentle reminder.

Give your evaluators as much help as possible. At the minimum, you will need to provide your personal statement and CV. If you have an unofficial transcript or the narrative evaluations from your clinical rotations, make those available as well. Provide a list of names and mailing addresses (in a neat and readable format) to the faculty member and his or her office staff.

One issue that is not resolved is that of access to your letter. The ERAS system, and local school policy in many cases, will ask you to choose between your right to view your letters and waiving this access. Your decision is often indicated in the letters or in other materials. If you are given this option, should you choose to view or waive? The argument for viewing your recommendations is that you gain control and the ability to suppress or modify a less than extraordinary letter. The argument for waiving your rights of access is that it allows and proclaims that the statements made in the letter are completely candid and, thus, presumably more reliable. Both assertions have merit. Unless you have significant reason to doubt your letter writer, waiving your rights is probably the better course. Choose your writers carefully and then give them the freedom to do their job. Ask that the letter writer include a statement at the end of the letter that you have waived your rights of access, and have them mail the letters directly to the programs you have specified. If your application will be electronic, the letter should be sent to your dean's office, which will scan them into the computer system.

The Dean's Letter

One letter you will not have to worry about is the dean's letter. This somewhat standardized letter is written by or for your dean's office and summarizes your medical school performance. It will recount your preclinical years, your performance on any licensure examinations ("Boards"), and the narrative comments made about you during your clinical rotations. These letters are not released to any program until November 1st each year. If you use the electronic application system, your dean's office will most likely scan your dean's letter into the ERAS system in advance of this date. Despite this, no program can view or print this information before November 1st.

Some schools will let you have a hand in developing the content of your dean's letter or will give you access to the contents after it is written. Just as with your rights of access to your individual letters of recommendation, the decision to view your dean's letter is a personal one. Many schools will ask you to meet with the dean or someone from the office who will be involved in generating the letter. This gives him or her a chance to get to know you and discuss the contents of your letter. If you have this opportunity, take it. This meeting will give you a chance to make the normally dry dean's letter much more personal. Because you are involved before the letter is written, you can still waive your rights of access, while remaining confident about the character of the letter.

Not every school invites your involvement in the dean's letter process. If you are concerned about the content of your dean's letter, make an appointment to meet with the appropriate person or persons who will compose the letter. Even if the school does not solicit your involvement, the dean may be more than happy for your input. If you are unsure of your school's practice, ask.

Final Hints

- Make friends with the office staff—they can be your best allies. They can help remind the busy faculty that their letter is due. They will be the ones who check the spelling and grammar. They will be the ones to put the letter on the correct letterhead. Don't overlook the vital role these people will play on your behalf.

- Allow sufficient time for your letters to be written. This means not only starting your portion of the process early, but giving the faculty lots of times to give your letter the attention it deserves. You will want all of your letter in the hands of the programs to which you are applying (or in the dean's office for ERAS applications) by November 1st—shoot for September 1st as your own target.
- Follow up on your requests. As the time draws near for you to submit your letters to the dean's office (for ERAS submission) or with your applications, check on the status of the letters. Don't make a pest of yourself, but do defend your needs for a timely letter.
- File only the letters the program requests. Although you have available more letters than you need, submit only the number each program requests. More letters will not make for a stronger application, it just increases the work of the selection committee and makes them wonder if your application needs extra help.
- A tactful way of getting to see your letters of recommendation (if you have not waived your rights of access) is to ask for a copy for your files. This will also give you an extra copy that you can send out later if you add a program to your application list. If this happens, you should always do your letter writers the courtesy of telling them you have sent another copy.
- If you want to gauge the potential you might have for an excellent letter, ask the faculty member if he or she knows you well enough to be able to write a "really strong letter of recommendation." This can give your potential letter writer a tactful way out and you can judge his or her level of enthusiasm before you make a final choice.

Chapter 12
Making the List—Theirs
(The Interview and After)

Getting the Slot

One of the most important hurdles that you must pass is getting an interview. While no one else will say it directly, if you don't have an interview, you don't have a chance. Even if you were the most desirable candidate a program ever had an application from, without some evidence of interest from you (in the form of an interview) the program will not rank you. The invitation for an interview is also an indication that you are considered competitive for the residency program. Given this importance, how do you go about getting the invitation?

The first task is obvious but still important; be sure your application is complete and submitted on time. Without this, you will not have a file with your desired program. Few programs will offer interviews before the receipt of the dean's letters, which are released November 1st. That does not mean that you wait until Thanksgiving to begin the process. Most programs will interview ten to twenty or more candidates for each position they have. Consequently, if you are serious about a program, make contact in early to mid-October to make sure that the program has begun receiving materials about you. Check to be sure that it has received your application and that some or all of your individual letters of recommendation have been received. [If you are using the electronic resident application system (ERAS), you can verify the generation of these letters by checking with the office at your own institution that puts them into your electronic file.] This not only ensures that your application is in the pipeline, but it begins to give you some measure of name recognition with the program. You become familiar with the key secretarial and office staff and they begin to know you as well. Ask when they may be making decisions about interview dates. How many dates will they have? Have the dates been set yet? When can you call to request an interview? Keep track of these answers and act quickly when the time comes to secure a spot. Generally, the onus is on you to obtain the interview.

Interview Timing

There are no good rules about the timing of interviews. Some argue that you should have your interview early in the season when both you and the interviewers are fresh. Others suggest later in the cycle (early January) so that you are fresh in the interviewers' minds when it comes time for them to make of their match list. Some mixture of the two is probably the most reasonable. You should probably plan on ten to fifteen interviews, so keep this in mind when your are working out the logistics.

If your medical school offers a residency in your chosen field, seriously consider applying and interviewing early with them even if you think you want to be moving on. This interview can serve to acquaint you with the process and give you experience before you set out to impress the folks at your ideal location. The faculty at your own school knows you well already so that a few fluffs will not harm your impression or chances. If you have a mentor who is part of the interview process, he or she may even be able to give you hints before or feedback after, but don't ask your mentor to compromise his or her role as interviewer by extending special favors. If your local program is one that you highly prize, you might substitute another regional program to serve a similar test-run function. With a test run or two behind you, you are ready for the heavyweights on your list. Remember that even Broadway plays go through out-of-town tryouts before they open.

The bulk of your interviews should be scheduled for late October to mid-November. (Some programs will offer an interview to internal candidates before the dean's letters are released.) Once you get in to the period from Thanksgiving to New Year's, travel becomes more difficult and people are more distracted. After New Year's, there are still interview slots, but many programs feel (rightly or wrongly) that the best candidates have already been through interviews there. There is a bias that these later candidates are inherently less well organized and motivated. While good candidates and eventual matches do come from this pool, waiting until January gives you less room for solving weather delays, finding missing letters of reference, or getting telephone calls of support.

If you have a spouse or significant other who will be moving with you and will be seeking employment, you will want to consider interviews for him or her as well. You may contact possible future employers directly or ask the program director's office staff if they have suggestions for possible employers in your partner's field. Even if your partner will not be working, strongly consider having him or her come along during the interview process. While you are interviewing, your partner can scout out the city, make inquiries about the reputation of the hospital or department, and begin to get a sense of the housing situation. Often just having someone to bounce ideas and observations off of at the end of the interview can help to solidify your impressions. A partner can also provide another perspective that can be helpful. Ultimately, you will not be happy in your new location if you partner is miserable.

Travel Tips

The process of interviewing is expensive in terms of both time and money. You can minimize the impact in a number of ways (Table 13-1).

Table 13-1. Travel Strategies

- Drive to interviews whenever possible and consider a carpool if several of your classmates are going to interview at the same institution.
- If your car is not reliable, consider renting a car. Rental cars are newer and in good repair. Do not assume that the rental car company's "corporate rate" is the best. The company's frequent renters are offered this rate, but it may be twice as much as a weekend or other special rate. Ask about special rates, promotions, or discounts. Some organizations (including the AAA, AMA, state medical societies, and many specialty societies) offer member discounts. Ask.
- Be aware that some car rental companies will not guarantee a reservation using a debit card (the kind that withdraws directly from you bank account.) Those that will accept this kind of card will put a hold on your account for more than the anticipated bill, which could leave you unexpectedly short if you go to write a check or visit an ATM in a strange city.
- If you are driving, plan your trip so you will not be traveling to or through deserted areas late at night.
- Get as many interviews as possible scheduled one after another in the same general region.
- If you are applying for a specialty position, try to schedule the interviews for both the preliminary and advanced position at the same time. Most institutions can accommodate this request.
- Use friends or family as a base of operations to save on hotel costs. This is less expensive and can pass for a family visit.
- Check with the institution to see if it has dormitory or other housing available at little or no cost. If not, the staff may be able to recommend inexpensive, nearby options. Unless you personally know the area, ask the staff for suggestions to avoid unsafe or substandard accommodations. You won't do your best if you were up all night watching the door or listening to police radios.
- Book airline travel well in advance to reduce the cost of tickets, and spend a Saturday night when possible to save even more. (The savings are often more than enough to pay for the hotel and meal expenses and give you more time to learn about the city.)
- Plan your travel to allow for unexpected delays and last-minute changes in plans. Don't forget that if you travel by air and have interviews in northern locations, weather in December and January can foil the best plans.

- Check with on-line services to get the best airfares and don't forget the low-cost carriers—you sacrifice amenities, but you still get there.
- While you will need cash for cab fare and incidentals, place all other services on credit cards to reduce your need for cash. You can delay credit card payments and the receipts provide documentation for tax purposes.

When you make your plans, check with the program staff to see if they have anything planned for the evening before the official interview schedule. Many programs offer informal mixers at the institution or in a faculty home. These functions are an excellent opportunity to see the program at a relaxed moment. You can talk candidly with the faculty and residents with whom you would work. You can get a sense of style, morale, and character. You will have to be on your best behavior, though, because they are getting to know you as well.

You should plan adequate time to arrive at the interview well in advance of the appointed starting time. This allows for unfamiliar traffic patterns, parking vagaries, and ambiguous hospital signage. I know of one candidate who arrived for a day's interview program two hours late, her attire was sloppy, and she gave no explanation. The candidate might just have well have sent her application to the dead-letter office.

The Required Suit (Clothes and Grooming)

It is a rite of fall to see flocks of navy-suited candidates, all bearing the look of deer during hunting season, wandering around the halls of hospitals and universities across the land. Does this mean that you must acquire the look of a Wall Street trainee when your tastes run more toward the Gap? Not exactly. You do have to remember that the more senior members of the interview team have weak hearts and strong feelings; it is best not to stress either.

For men, the options are mercifully simple: a seasonally appropriate suit, or sport jacket with neutral slacks, will always fit the bill. (Seersucker in January will not work at even the most "Southern" of your choices.) Jackets should be buttoned, though they may be opened when sitting. Your shirt should be a tastefully muted, clean, pressed, and long-sleeved. White or blue is the best color. Your tie (yes, you need one) may make a statement, but should not speak louder than you do. When in doubt, opt for the more conservative. A washable tie will reduce the chance of making a spot bigger should a spill occur. At one time, hair length was an issue. Now the choice is more open, but it should be clean, well managed, and not too far from the mainstream.

Women have a harder time because their options are greater. The tailored business suit will work as well as tasteful day wear. A pants suit would be fine. You do not have to opt for navy or black. The color should be chosen to complement your coloring and style, but should be muted in tone. Provocative or casual dress is as out of place as an open collar is for a man. You should choose conservative makeup for day wear, not evening wear. Hairstyles are as varied as the individual, and you will be the best judge of what works for you. As with men, neatness and cleanliness count.

Jewelry (for both sexes) should be tasteful and understated. The balance must be between demonstrating appropriate attention to detail and suggesting obsessive narcissism. When in doubt, less is better. Your own style and judgment can still be evident, just quietly stated. You want to make a pleasant statement, not shout at the top of your lungs "look at me." You will be hired for your interest and abilities. Extremes will attract the wrong type of attention. (They can find out about the nose ring after you have the position.)

For both sexes, shoes should be leather and clean, if not freshly polished. You will be walking quite a bit between hospital tours, interview offices, and other locations, so make sure that your shoes are comfortable. Hands and nails should be clean and well kept. Perfume, cologne, and after-shave should be omitted. (You don't want to be remembered for the allergic reaction of the chief resident.) Gum chewing can help keep you awake while you are driving, but should be off limits during the interview. Some quick clothing and travel tips are included in Table 13-2.

Table 13-2. Travel tips

- Hang out your suit and shirt or blouse the night before to allow some of the wrinkles to disappear. Hanging them in the bathroom when you take your shower will speed the process even more.
- Pack light: make the most of items that can be mixed and matched to form new looks from the same pallet of choices. Remember that each location will not compare notes (about dress at least) with your next stop, so outfits can be reused if they are still clean and presentable.
- If you travel by plane and can easily get your things into a manageable carry-on bag, do so. The airlines cannot lose a bag you carry yourself. The bag must meet the airline's rules as to size, shape, and weight, and you must be able to lift it. Remember that you may have to carry it between two airport gates that have different zip codes.
- Pick outfits (for either gender) that have pockets. These are invaluable for carrying airline tickets, change for parking meters and pay phones, hotel keys, emergency cash, professors' names, office phone numbers, and the like. For women, pockets may allow you to reduce the size or even the need for a purse, greatly simplifying your life.
- Pack for a range of weather and events. If one or more of your interview stops will include an informal get-together, pack to allow a casual option.
- Take a folding umbrella and some stain remover.
- Save one or two of those little bottles of hotel shampoo and reuse them to carry a small amount of laundry soap for those unexpected spills and last minute detox missions.

- A package of breath mints can give you confidence as well as better breath. Remember that foil wrapped ones will set off the metal detectors in most airports, so take them out of your pocket before you go through.
- Because most of your visits will occur during the cold and flu season, you should carry a pocket-sized package of tissues or several tissues from the hotel, neatly folded. Medications for the symptoms of these infections are a reasonable addition to your travel supplies, but avoid those that sedate.

Sparkling

You are selling yourself during the interview. This is your chance to show them your personality, which cannot be conveyed in a résumé. How do you set yourself apart from the other candidates who will be interviewing at any given program? You do it with "sparkle." Think about the times that you met extraordinary people. What made them unforgettable, engaging, special? Odds are that it was that hard-to-define characteristic, sparkle. They were probably animated, interested and interesting, a good listener as well as a lively conversationalist. They were probably knowledgeable, well rounded, and sophisticated. They were articulate and insightful, but not self-absorbed, pretentious, or pompous. They probably had a sense of humor, but knew how to temper its use.

It does not take a Dale Carnegie course in personality to develop your own version of sparkle. You should not try to be someone or something you are not. However, this is not the time to be a passive participant either. Be animated, but relax and be yourself. Let your interviewer know you are excited to be there for the interview. Ask questions, and really listen to the answers. Show that you have an interest in the interviewer and the program. Make your interviewers feel like they are not just stop number twelve on your interview migration, but don't try to make them believe that they are the only object of your pilgrimage either. They know better. It is O.K. to use your hands as long as your palms are dry and you don't knock anything over. While it is important to be lively and observe your surroundings, do not forget the importance of eye contact.

In preparation for the interview trail, try sitting in front of a mirror and assessing your posture, demeanor, and hand placement. This will give you an idea of the image you are presenting. Do you present the image of someone you would want to meet or get to know better? If not, what would change that? Do remember, that flirting, with or by either sex, is strictly out of bounds.

Fielding Questions

You will certainly be asked questions as a part of the interview—that is the nature of the process. Your answers should be straightforward, to the point, and preferably short. If you are unsure or do not know, say so. That is better than faking it. Do keep your answers consistent; several people may ask you the same question and they may compare answers later. Do not expect clinical questions in your chosen field. While these do sometimes show up, seasoned interviewers know that they will have many years to teach you these things and you should not be expected to know the information now. (If such a question is asked, the interviewer is probably just trying to see how you tackle a problem, so answer accordingly. Profess your inexperience and lack of knowledge, relate to a similar patient you have seen, or turn it around to find out how the problem is managed in that institution.)

There are a number of questions that can be anticipated well in advance of any interview (Table 13-3). Sometimes questions are asked not for the content of your response but for your style. For example: What do you think of managed care? What do you think of global warming? Gene splicing? The Internet? Abortion? Supply-side economics? Postmodern films? The questioner does not expect you to have solved world hunger or the riddle of the Gordian Knot. They do want to know if you recognize that the latter is not an Edwardian method of tying a man's tie. Have you thought about some of the more weighty questions of our time and medicine? Can you put forward a cogent argument? Can you look at both sides of an argument and critically evaluate the points expressed? A little advanced thought on some of these questions will keep you from being caught flat-footed by the question. "Glazed" is not a bad attribute for donuts; it is bad for residency candidates.

Table 13-3. Common Questions for Interviewees

Why did you choose medicine?
Why did you choose this field for your career? What do you like about it? What do you dislike?
Why did you choose this institution to apply to? What attracted you to us? What do you want from a residency? From this residency?
What do you see yourself doing at the end of residency? Practice? Teaching? Research? Industry?
If your CV lists employment or research experience, what was your role? What did you learn from the experience?
What do you think are your greatest personal strengths? What are your greatest weaknesses? What strengths do you bring to residency?
How would you classify your personality? How would someone else classify it? What are your strengths and weaknesses in dealing with people?
Have you ever had to make a decision you knew would be unpopular or would hurt someone else? Have you ever faced an ethical dilemma? How did you resolve it?

What do you think someone else would say was your style of leadership? How
  do you resolve conflicts? What frustrates you? What motivates you? How
  do you solve problems?
Is there anything in your life you wish you could do over, and why?
What hobbies do you have? How do you like to relax?
What was the last (nontechnical) book you read? The last movie you saw? How
  did you like them?
In what area of the country did you grow up? Do you have family in this
  geographic area?
If you have a family, how would they feel about moving to this area? If you are
  married, engaged, or involved, have you considered work options for your
  significant other?

Getting Information

The interview process is a two-way interaction: you are interviewing them at the
same time they are interviewing you. Do your homework before you start on
your quest. As discussed in Chapters 4 and 7, you need to have some form of
file or database on the programs you are considering. Review your records
looking for both missing information and areas that are fertile for discussion. Do
you know the programs' policy on meeting attendance? Do they provide
disability insurance? How often do they have visiting speakers at their
departmental meetings? How accessible are the departmental luminaries? What
expectations or opportunities are there for research?

     During your meeting with the selection committee, be alert to opportunities
to take a topic raised by the interviewer and extend the dialogue with your own
question. This should be a logical extension of the discussion and not forced, but
many subjects will provide obvious jumping-off points. For example: If you are
asked about your hobbies, feel free to ask about options for exploring your pet
passion. Ask how the interviewers thinks *your* strengths (that you just
enumerated) might fit with the strengths of *their* residency program. Ask the
resident giving your tour of the facilities if he or she has a chance to interact
with the department's luminaries or if they are always out of town or
unapproachable. Do not be afraid to ask the same questions of several different
people during your visit; you may get different answers from the residents and
faculty. Do not shy away from pointed questions; if it needs to be asked, ask.
Some ideas for questions that you might ask are given in Table 13-4.

Table 13-4. Common questions for you to ask

What are the strengths and weaknesses of the program? How does it compare to other programs in the area, region, or nation?
How do residents do on national in-training examinations? How do graduates do on certification examinations once they complete the program?
Do residents go on to fellowships? If so, how many and where?
What didactic programs are give by the department? Is the time protected so that you can attend?
Do all the faculty participate in teaching? If not, who carries the greatest share?
What special resident benefits are offered that are not offered at other programs?
What is the night call system like? Does it work well? Is there adequate time for families and reading?
Have there been any changes in faculty in the past year or two? Are there any planned or known? Is the leadership of the program and department stable? Personable? Approachable? Accessible?
Have any residents left the program before graduation? If so, why?
Is there good camaraderie in the department? Among the faculty? Within the resident staff?
Are the faculty respected? By the residents? By the outside world?

Just as you have to watch the body-language signals you are sending, you should be an astute observer of the interviewer's demeanor as well. Do all the residents you meet look exhausted, depressed, and undernourished? Do they grumble or bubble? Do they smile at you and each other? When you sit in the chairman's outer office waiting to meet, is the tenor of the office rushed and stressed, or relaxed and friendly? You can get a lot of information about the place by just watching. They are watching you; it is only fair that you do the same.

After the Interview

When the day's schedule of meetings, dialogues, handshakes, tours, and thank yous are over, what then? As we will discuss in the next chapter, your tasks are just beginning. Before your day is complete and you move on (physically and to the next chapter) there are a couple of things to consider. If you do not have tight flight connections or a long drive ahead of you, ask if you can go with one of the residents to a clinic, the operating room, a lecture, or the departmental library. (The do have one, don't they?) Wander to the cafeteria, the gift shop, or the front entrance, and people watch for a few minutes. What are the patients, visitors, employees, and house staff like? How busy do the emergency room or the clinics appear to be? Is the building clean and well maintained? These factors will contribute to your overall impression of the place and will determine the desirability of spending the next few years of your life in this institution.

Before you depart, ask whether you are expected to communicate again with the program before the match. Some programs or program directors expect you to contact them if you remain interested in the program; others do not. It is best to know the expectations of the program before you leave. Even if a program does not expect follow-up communications, a personal thank you note (hand written if you have good handwriting) is always a good idea. It reinforces your name and interest. You can even use it to reiterate some of your strengths and why you are a good fit to this particular program. Don't overdo this part, let your personal statement and letters of recommendation do it for you.

Secret Tips

Here are some additional "secret" tips to help with the interview process:

- Practice interviews can give valuable experience and insight into the process, relieving some of the tension and making you more polished. An alternative to the practice interview is a mock interview before you ever head out on the interview trail. This may be offered by members of the faculty of your medical school, a mentor (if you have one), other classmates, or even a friend or spouse. You can easily envision the types of questions that might come up or you would ask if the roles were reversed. These can form the basis of a mock interview. If you want more help with the process, the Resources section at the end of this book lists a number of books on interviews and interviewing.
- Unless you have a poor memory, do not try to take notes during the actual interview. Notes immediately after are a good idea; notes during are a distraction for both you and the other person.
- Always be considerate, respectful, and courteous to the administrative staff you encounter before, during, or after your interview. A negative comment from an offended staff member can demolish an otherwise promising career.
- When introduced to someone, a firm, self-assured handshake is appropriate for both men and women. This should not be the death grip of a pro wrestler, nor should it be the tentative dead fish of your great aunt at a funeral. With this simple gesture, you convey confidence, pride, and poise. Right or wrong, it provides a sense of honesty, integrity, and trustworthiness, although there should be no logical relationship to these qualities. When combined with a smile, this is a great way to make the all-important first impression.

- If your hands are cold or your palms sweaty, put them under your coat, in a pocket, or under the edge of your thigh while you wait. This both dries and warms them before you have to shake hands.
- To avoid the appearance of fatigue late in the day, a lunchtime beverage with caffeine may help, but remember that caffeine stimulates diuresis and bladder tone. The choice is yours, but consider both the pros and cons carefully.
- Even if you normally have wine with your meal, avoid alcohol during the interview process. It may impair your sleep the night before and certainly may affect both image and performance if ordered during lunch.
- You're a damn fool if you curse during the interview.

Chapter 13
After the Interview

The interview is over; you have survived another one. That is one major hurtle out of the way, but the job is not over yet. Several essential things must still happen. You have to collect your thoughts, wrap up loose ends, and begin to think about what you saw. These elements are just as important, though less pressing, than what has gone before.

Like you, the program selection committee will have a number of things that must be accomplished in the hours, days, and weeks that follow your visit. You both must assess the interview and its results. You will need to evaluate each other's strengths and weaknesses, and keep some record of the outcomes. Each may want to convey their interest in the other as part of the courting ritual that is the match. Each of these elements brings you both closer to a true match.

What They Do After You Leave

After the interviews of the day are finished, some or all of the faculty and residents will get together to form a composite evaluation. This is usually made up of those who were part of the formal interview team, but may also include members of the department who were less active participants in the process. Residents who gave the tour, those who took the candidates to lunch, and the person who introduced the city or program may all contribute their observations. If the program has a get-together the evening before, those who met you there may be included. This should alert you to be on your best behavior for your entire stay.

When the interview team or selection committee meets, the candidates are given some form of ranking score. No matter the form, this score is designed to help compare the students when the last candidate has been interviewed, sometimes months later. Your qualifications will certainly be part of this, but other aspects carry as much or even more weight. Your long-term plans, family considerations, demeanor, drive, personality, candidness, and other impressions all play a part. The interview team may have had a series of questions or areas of discussion that more than one interviewer covered. If this is the case, your responses will be compared.

Some time in January, there is a final caucus involving the entire department. At this meeting, the applicant's portfolio is evaluated again and comparisons are made with other candidates with similar scores. Follow-up from the applicants, experience with them during a rotation, and other factors may move the applicant up or down the list. Contact from you indicating your interest, messages of support from faculty, or even a thank-you note can influence the results of this final caucus.

While not all programs will do so, some programs will send candidates a letter or telephone them to indicate the program's interest in them as a future resident. If this happens, it is a good sign that you are competitive and the program is interested. The absence of such an indication does not mean that the program is not interested. It may not give an indication to anyone. This varies from program to program and hospital to hospital. Be forewarned that the statements you and the program make about rankings are nonbinding when it comes time to make the rank order list.

Notes to Yourself

One of the first things for you to do, on the plane, in the hotel, or when you get back home, is to make notes to yourself about what you saw, and the impressions you had. This is the time to fill in any blanks in your information database (Figure 13-1). Did you find out about parking or a book allowance? What is their policy on paternity leave? How would you rank resident morale and cohesiveness? If you don't have your database with you on your travels, use the hotel stationery, envelopes, or even paper towels, but get the notes down. Hospitals are remarkably similar (ask anyone who has visited more than one Veterans Administration hospital), so confusion is easy. Several months after the interview, it may be impossible to place the program that you liked so much, (you know, the one with the blue tile walls) without notes to yourself.

Immediately after the interview is a good time to review the important deadlines and contact information. If the department chairman or program director has changed, make sure you update your records. It is not good form to address something to the former chairman. Make note of any follow-up that is expected by the program; some programs request it, others don't want it. (If follow-up is in order, don't forget to put a reminder on your calendar of events so it does not get overlooked in the last days of the process.)

Evaluation Checklist

Program Name: _____

Program Director: _____

Working Rank: [   ]

Interview date: _____

Notes

Program

- Conferences
- Core teaching
- Electives
- Evaluations
- Research requirement
- Scut
- Subspecialty options

Grade _____

Patient care

- Adequate supervision
- Consultations
- Continuity of care
- Exposure to private patients
- Graded responsibility
- Quantity of cases
- Quality of cases
- Subspecialty exposure
- Teaching expected

Grade _____

Faculty

- Number
- Availability
- Educational interest
- Diversity
- Rapport
- Subspecialty interest

Grade _____

House staff

- Number
- Departures
- Morale
- Peer relationships
- Plans: Academic
          Practice
          Research

Grade _____

Facilities

- Buildings
- Call rooms
- Clinics
- Operating rooms

Grade _____

Notes

Library / Support

- Accessibility / hours
- Book & journal selection
- Computers
- Internet access
- Secretarial support
- Slide-making facilities

Grade _____

Benefits

- Days off
- Education
- Maternity / Paternity
- Sickness
- Vacation
- Insurance
- Dental
- Disability
- Health
- Life
- Spouse coverage
- Malpractice
  - Amount
  - Tail   Yes   No
- Reimbursement
  - Books
  - Dues
  - Journals
  - Meetings
- Salary
- Copying
- Food allowance
- Laundry
- Uniforms
- Moonlighting

Grade _____

Community

- Climate
- Family
  - Education
  - Job
  - Proximity
  - Spouse
- Organization
- Housing
- Recreation

Grade _____

Figure 13-1 A simple check list will help to organize your thoughts about the programs you are considering.

This is also a good time to decide if you want to return for a follow-up visit. Not every program can accommodate such a request, and if you make such a visit, it must be as an observer following a resident through his or her day. This option should be reserved for only the most desirable and competitive programs on your list. It is time-consuming and generally will not significantly increase your competitiveness by much, if any. It will give you more information about the day-to-day functioning of the department, a sense of the resident's duties, and the flavor of the program. It may be worth the effort if you are uncertain.

Notes to Them

If you are interested in a particular program, a note from you expressing your interest is never out of place. This should be genuine and reserved for those programs that are truly near the top of your list. The note should be sent to the program director or the chairman of the department. It should be straightforward, to the point, and short (Figure 13-2). It may be typed, computer printed, or hand written, but if you go this latter route, it must be legible. If you go with a computer-printed letter, it should not sound like a mail-merge form and must be printed on a high quality-printer. The signature must always be original. The use of personal stationery is not necessary, though it can be a nice touch. If you have access to a computer, it is easy to create your own version of stationery (Figure 13-3a). If you go this route, less is more; avoid anything unprofessional, grandiose, or overblown (Figure 13-3b).

Whether a program requests some indication of your interest or not, a brief thank-you note will get you noticed and is worth the time. This note is best when hand written (legibly), but a neatly typed note will suffice if your handwriting is not the best. Notes should be sent to those with whom you most closely interacted or those who provided special help. Because these notes are usually included in your file, do not make each note the same as the last. You can customize each note with some special comment or thank you for something distinctive the person did or said (Figure 13-4a). Remember that it is better not to send a note than to send something that sounds insincere, illiterate, or like a template (Figure 13-4b). Just like in grade school, neatness counts.

November 28, 2000

Dr. John Dolittle
Program Director
The Residency
Old Pooh-Pooh University
Ocean View, Illinois, 61821

Dear Dr. Dolittle:

I wanted to tell you how much I enjoyed my visit to your program on the 23rd. The hospitality extended to me was greatly appreciated, as was all the information provided me about your program. I was very impressed by everything I saw and will be ranking your program very highly. I hope that your were also pleased with the attributes that I could bring to the program and will rank me favorably as well.

If I may provide any additional information to assist with your evaluation of my candidacy, I will be happy to provide them.

Sincerely yours,

Figure 13-2 If you use a computer to generate your thank-you letters, remember that the recipients may compare notes so vary your letters that are going to the same institution.

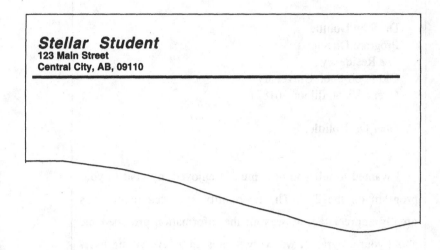

Figure 13-3a

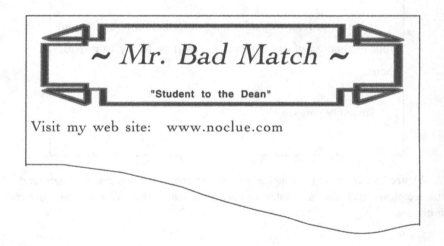

Figure 13-3b

There and many pros and cons behind the option of having a faculty member at your institution place a call to a friend at your most-coveted program. It lets your own program know that it is not necessarily your first choice, potentially limiting your fallback positions. It may seem to the recipient institution that you are over-eager or under-qualified. It does, however, have the potential to get you noticed when it is a truly personal friend-to-friend message. If you use this, use it sparingly and only when a true relationship between the involved faculty exists.

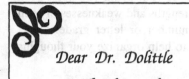

Dear Dr. Dolittle

Thank you for taking the time to tell me about the extensive historical library that is a part of your program. The availability of this kind of resourse is exactly what I am looking for in making my residency selections.

Thanks

Stellar Student

Figure 13-4a

Dear Sir:

Thanks for seeing me. I know I
will be the best resident you
ever seen.

Mr. Bad Match

Figure 13-4b

After the Last Interview

After your last interview is finished, it is time to review. Go back over the notes you made after each interview. Are there any loose ends to be taken care of? Have all your questions been answered? Have all of your thank-you notes been sent? Make notes to yourself about the relative strengths and weaknesses of each program (Figure 13-5). Give each program a number or letter grade. Don't worry, these scores are temporary; they are just to help organize your thoughts while your impressions are still fresh.

Program	Pros	Cons	Score
Pooh-Pooh U.	Famous Big Lots of patients	Hard to get into Limited contact with faculty	A

City Hospital	Serves the medically
	   needy
	Should be an easy
	   match (safety net)
		Faculty not well
		   known
		Safety of
		   neighborhood
		   unknown
		Not in good repair
			B

Regional Health Center	Intimate size
	Good contact with
	   faculty
	Good parking
		Not many unusual
		   cases
		Poor health plan
		Hard to get to, no
		   airport
			A

Community Health Partners	Private practice setting
	Personal attention
		No university
		   affiliation
		Not many teaching
		   conferences
			B+

Figure 13-5

As you develop your program appraisals, don't forget to get counsel from your advisor, spouse or significant other, parents, and friends. While the final assessment must be yours, discussing it with other people will force you to articulate your thoughts. They can help provide balance and perspective. Most importantly, if they will be a part of your move, their observations and concerns must be considered in the final ranking.

Now you are ready to begin the process of ranking your programs, and that is where we go next.

Chapter 14
Making the List—Your Match List

One of the greatest strengths of the matching process is its deference to the preferences of the student. The matching algorithm gives each student a match to the program on his or her list with highest possible ranking. Therefore, your list of programs, and the order in which you list them, is extremely important. While most of the hard part of the residency search process is behind you by the time you are ready to make your list, it is too early to become complacent. (You can do that the day after the match results are announced.)

The list we are referring to, called the Rank Order List or ROL, indicates to the matching system which programs you would consider, and what your order of preference would be. Candidate submit their list by way of the Internet using the Rank Order List and Input Confirmation (WebROLIC) system. This system was developed and implemented during the 1999 match cycle. Your list can contain preliminary, transitional, or specialty programs, depending on your situation and career path. These different types, and even different specialties, can be intermixed within your list. If you are applying for an advanced position (to start in the second postgraduate year) you will also submit a supplemental rank order list for the first year (preliminary) position that you will need. Worksheets for the rank order lists are available on-line from the NRMP Web site, although you do have to be registered for the match to access the appropriate area.

Which Ones?

One of the paramount rules of the matching system is that you should not put any program on your list if you would be unwilling to attend. The same rule applies to programs; if you are on their list, they have said they would be willing to accept you as a resident. The result of this mutual agreement is that you must only list programs that you found sufficiently desirable to commit to for the next several years.

Your list should include all of the programs that you feel you would be happy to be in, regardless of what you think your chances are of matching. You may have been told that you were the best candidate a particular program has ever interviewed, but don't count on matching there. Conversely, just because you did not get flowers and a note when you got home does not mean they don't want to see you again. Neither you nor the program is bound by anything that is said about specific ranking. While it is assumed that neither party will grossly lie, specifics about final ranking are privileged and unofficial until the list (yours and theirs) is filed. General statements are fair game and should be indicative of interest, but that is a long way from a specific rank number. (Note: it is against NRMP rules for a program to ask you how you will rank them—they can't ask, you don't have to tell.)

Because you do not know the final rank order used by each of the programs you applied to, and the programs do not know the candidates' lists, you both may be surprised by the outcome. Since the system attempts to get the student the best program possible, others ranked higher than you by the program may go elsewhere, leaving you a spot despite not being first in line. This is the time to vote your true feelings and not worry about what the program may do.

As you decide if a program is an acceptable one, go back over your notes—you know, the ones you were supposed to make right after the interview? Look at your overall impressions. Do you see yourself fitting in with the department? Did it share your style? What is the quality of the educational experience? How well will the program prepare you for the career you envision? What are the strengths and weaknesses of the program and how do these compare to other programs you visited? These questions will help you not only decide if the program should stay on your "A" list, but may also begin to suggest a hierarchy that will help when it comes time to do the Rank Order List.

How Many?

Your decision about the number of programs to rank has already been partially made, when you decided on the number of programs to apply to (Chapter 2). For obvious reasons, this number represents the maximum number of programs you can list. Additionally, there is little point of ranking any program that did not grant you an interview, further reducing the pool from which to choose. (Keep these extra programs in mind in case you have to face the scramble.) These two factors set the upper boundary, but what is a functional number to rank?

To reduce the chances of being unmatched, you should list all of the programs that you have applied to that would be acceptable residency positions. But what about those extra ones? It would seem that while it is extraordinarily unlikely that a program will rank you if you have not had an interview, why not rank them all, as long as you applied? (There is, after all, no penalty for listing these programs, although there is a $30 per ranking for each program above fifteen.) For practical purposes, this is not a good strategy to avoid the scramble (it is unlikely to work and it can get very expensive). You should be realistic with your list.

Unless you are a Nobel laureate, listing less than half the number of programs to which you applied, or virtually all the programs you interviewed with, is suggestive of suicidal ideation. With no enforceable promises or way to assure your chances at the various programs, it is foolhardy to list only your top choices. The only exception might be the extraordinarily qualified student who is seeking a position is a less competitive field. Do not go this route without careful counsel from your advisor. The bottom line: list every program where you interviewed and that you would be willing to go to for residency. Certainly, you should not list any program that you could not be delighted with if you were extended a contract. This is true even if you were assured in writing that the program was going to rank you "number one" on its Rank Order List. If you wouldn't go to the program, it is better to seek a position in the scramble than be forced to be miserable for the next years of your life at a program you hate.

Because of the cost structure, and the realities of application and interviewing, the practical limit to the number of programs students will rank is fifteen. For most students, this matches well with the above guidelines. Nationally, the average number of programs ranked is over seven and in the last round of the match (1999), roughly 80% of matched students matched to one of their top three choices (Figure 14-1). The NRMP has collected data for the last four years on the relationship between the average length of the Rank Order Lists of matched applicants and filled programs vs. the average length of lists of unmatched applicants and unfilled programs. Reviewing the data shows that there is a consistent pattern of matched applicants and filled programs having longer ROLs than unmatched students and unfilled programs (Table 14-1). (The average program that fills will list almost nine students per slot they fill, while programs that do not fill average fewer than five students.)

Who Goes First?

This question is easy. The answer, however, can be difficult. The Rank Order List should always reflect your true assessment of desirability of the various programs and should never be based on any other considerations. What is difficult is codifying the factors that go into this assessment. For most students, the final determination will be based on intangibles: It just feels right. Factors such as geography, family considerations, educational strength, and reputation will all factor in. While is it perfectly acceptable to get suggestions from significant others, your advisor, or even family, the final choice must be yours, and you are not obligated to share the results of that choice with anyone. Just like the preference for a color of an automobile, or the preference for sushi, lots of people will have opinions, but only yours will count.

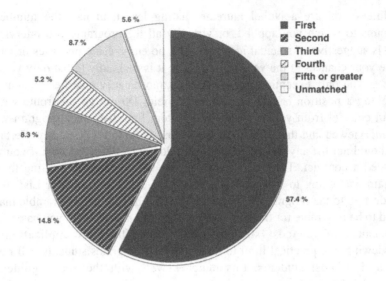

Figure 14-1 In 1999, over 57% of United States applicants matched to their first choice, while only 6% remained unmatched.

Table 14-1 Average Length of Rank Order Lists for Matched and Unmatched Candidates

Year	Matched Applicants		Unmatched Applicants	
	Matched	Average ROLs	Unmatched	Average ROLs
1996	17,404 (73.3%)	6.43	6,337 (26.7%)	5.38
1997	17,616 (69.6%)	6.89	7,686 (30.4%)	5.16
1998	17,698 (69.8%)	7.32	7,674 (30.2%)	4.95
1999	17,873 (70.4%)	7.42	7,519 (29.6%)	5.06

(Data from National Residency Matching Program, used with permission.)

As noted before, you will use the WebROLIC system to enter you Rank Order List. There is no provision for submitting your list as a paper copy or as an e-mail; it must be submitted by way of the NRMP Web page using your NRMP code number and personal identification number (PIN). You do not have to enter the list all at once and you may make changes to your list, right up to the deadline. Each year, the NRMP announces the starting and ending date for this process (usually early in January and the second week in February, respectively). Before the starting date, you can, and should, print out a ROL worksheet that you can use to develop and keep track of your preferences. Once the start date has passed, you can go to the Web site and enter your list.

It is best to enter your Rank Order List well in advance of the deadline. This allows time for you to have second thoughts (you probably will) and insures against slow response times, a sluggish Web, or a computer crash at the last minute. At 11:59 p.m. (Eastern Time) on the day of the deadline, all lists are frozen, no exceptions. (Don't forget to correct for the time difference in your area if you end up with a last-minute dash to the computer lab.)

The Safety Net

Some students regard the less competitive residencies on their list as a "safety net." These programs are acceptable but less desirable to the student, and are ones with a high likelihood of a match. This type of Rank Order List entry does reduce your chances of remaining unmatched and there is little reason not to include them unless they would cause a financial hardship because of the increased listing fee.

As you prepare your final list, take a good look to decide about the need for your plan B. If you ended up with a very short list, or if you are seeking a place in a very competitive field, you may want to add some of the backup programs you had applied to as a contingency. As with so much of the process, seek the advice of your advisor before you decide to either add or skip your safety net programs.

Chapter 15

Special Circumstances

As we have noted before, most students seeking a residency position in the United States go through the NRMP process. There are, however, some situations and exceptions that modify the process: If you are looking for a career in neurology, neurosurgery, ophthalmology, otolaryngology, or urology, you will participate in your own specialty matching process. The residency programs offered by the various branches of the military have a separate matching process, as do programs in Canada or those specific to osteopathic medical students. The special needs of couples who wish to match together provide another set of opportunities and problems that carry their own set of nuances. Understanding how these particulars change the process allows you to turn special circumstances into special opportunities.

Military Programs

The uniformed services (Army, Navy, and Air Force) residencies have their own version of the matching process. Anyone can apply to these programs and participate in the military match as long as they would qualify for commission in the armed forces. Most candidates in this process will be graduates of the Uniformed Services University of Health Sciences Medical School or will have participated in the Health Professions Scholarship programs. These students have a military service obligation and will generally have priority in the match. The military match process involves interviews and selections that occur earlier in the year than the NRMP match process. Consequently, decisions (and announcements) are made well before the NRMP match day. Because match rates vary widely from service to service and specialty to specialty, it is best to register for the NRMP matching process at the same time. The NRMP requires that if you are matched through the military matching program, you must immediately withdraw from the NRMP. The deadline for this withdrawal is the same as the deadline for the submission or Rank Order Lists and is well after the announcement of the military match results. For more specifics on the mechanics of this process, or to obtain application materials, contact your local Armed Services recruiter.

Specialty Matches

A number of advanced specialties carry out separate matches that are managed by either the NRMP (orthopedics, cardiovascular medicine, gastroenterology, infectious disease, and pulmonary disease), a separate matching service (ophthalmology, otolaryngology, neurology, neurosurgery, and plastic surgery), or the specialty itself (urology). Additionally, there are separate matching processes for advanced fellowship training programs that go beyond the scope of this book.

Medical Specialties and Orthopedics

The Medical Specialty Matching Service (MSMP) offered by the NRMP functions exactly like the general match with three exceptions: There are a different set of deadlines, Rank Order Lists are submitted by mail and you will have to submit a supplemental Rank Order List for the associated preliminary slot. The NRMP provides lists of programs and information on its Internet site in much the same way that it does for the general match (Figure 15-1).

To participate in the MSMP, you have to submit a supplemental Rank Order List for your preliminary program and a separate (paper) Rank Order List for the specialty match. There is a $40 fee to participate in the specialty match. More importantly, there is a different set of deadlines to keep track of as you go through the process (Table 15-1). You will have to watch the dates for both the regular match (for the preliminary position) and the specialty match, so be careful.

Table 15-1

December	Agreements available for programs and students
Late May	Programs and students must file to be listed in the materials supplied by the MSMP
Late April	Rank Order List forms mailed
Mid- to late May	**Deadline** for receipt or Rank Order Lists from both programs and applicants (date varies slightly for medical specialties and orthopedics—check.)
Early June	Match results announced for orthopedics
Mid-June	Match results announced for medical specialties

MSMP Program Directory
2000 Positions

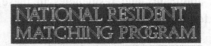

NATIONAL RESIDENT
MATCHING PROGRAM

NRMP Home   AAMC Home

Hospitals are listed alphabetically by city within state.

A program's CODE is used by applicants to list that program on their Rank Order Lists.

A program's QUOTA is the number of positions offered in the Match by that program.

CARDIOVASCULAR DISEASE

ALABAMA

```
UNIVERSITY OF SOUTH ALABAMA
CARDIOLOGY FELLOWSHIP PROGRAM
2451 FILLINGIM STREET
MOBILE, AL 36617
Telephone: (334) 471-7923
     Program Description        Code  Quota
     CARDIOVASCULAR DISEASE     326171    1
     Program Director: VASKAR MUKERJI MD
```

ARIZONA

```
CARDIOLOGY FELLOWSHIP PROGRAM
1111 E MCDOWELL ROAD
PHOENIX, AZ 85006
Telephone: (602) 239-6743
     Program Description        Code  Quota
     CARDIOVASCULAR DISEASE     111171    3
     Program Director: KENNETH B DESSER MD
```

```
UNIV OF ARIZONA COLL OF MED
CARDIOLOGY FELLOWSHIP PROGRAM
1501 N CAMPBELL  ROOM 6402
TUCSON, AZ 85724
Telephone: (520) 626-6221
     Program Description        Code  Quota
     CARDIOLOGY 3YR             112271    2
     Program Director: G EWY MD/W ROESKE MD
```

Figure 15-1 The Medical Specialty Matching Program (MSMP) functions like its parent, the NRMP, with similar information but slightly modified processes. (From National Residency Matching Program, used with permission.)

One difference between the general match and the specialty matches operated through the MSMP is the method used to announce the results. On the date the results are released, they are sent by overnight courier to the programs and to unmatched applicants. Matched applicants have their information sent at the same time, but it is sent by first-class mail, and arrives later, giving a unmatched students a chance to "scramble" for unfilled positions.

The San Francisco Match

Students interested in careers in ophthalmology, otolaryngology, neurology, neurosurgery, and plastic surgery use a matching service called the San Francisco Matching Programs (Figure 15-2). This privately run matching service connects applicants and residencies in these fields and coordinates (some) specialty fellowship assignments.

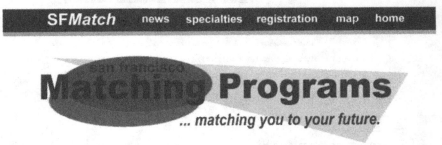

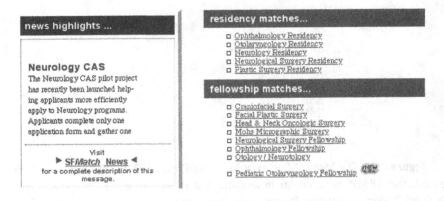

Figure 15-2 The San Francisco Matching Programs service offers a matching service for students interested in programs in ophthalmology, otolaryngology, neurology, neurosurgery, and plastic surgery. (Used with permission of the San Francisco Matching Programs.)

Like the Medical Specialties Matching Program of the NRMP, the San Francisco match has its own set of application deadlines and announcement dates (Figure 15-3). Like the MSMP, this means that you have to juggle two sets of matching processes as you compete, using the NRMP for your preliminary training and this system for your advanced training.

Residency Matches: *(See bottom of page for key to this chart)*

Specialty (Subspecialty to Register)	Match Deadline (Rank lists due)	Results Released (Program/Direct Entry/ranking)	Applicant Results (Applicant's entry notification)	Vacancies Released (Announcement, vacant and waiting lists)	Training Begins (Year by which training begins)
Otolaryngology, PGY-2	Monday Jan 10, 2000	Friday Jan 21, 2000	Tuesday Jan 25, 2000	Monday Jan 31, 2000	2001
Ophthalmology, PGY-2	Monday Jan 17, 2000	Friday Jan 28, 2000	Tuesday Feb 1, 2000	Monday Feb 7, 2000	2001
Neurology, PGY-2	Monday Jan 17, 2000	Friday Jan 28, 2000	Tuesday Feb 1, 2000	Monday Feb 7, 2000	2000 / 2001
Neurosurgery, PGY-2	Monday Jan 24, 2000	Wednesday Feb 2, 2000	Friday Feb 4, 2000	Monday Feb 14, 2000	2001
Plastic Surgery, PGY-4	Monday May 15, 2000	Monday May 22, 2000	Wednesday May 24, 2000	Monday May 29, 2000	2001

Figure 15-3 The timetable for the San Francisco match varies slightly for each specialty. This is the timetable for the 2000 match. (Used with permission of the San Francisco Matching Programs.)

The San Francisco Matching Program has recently developed a Central Application Service (CAS) that is similar in concept to the ERAS system (Figure 15-4). With this system, the candidate fills out one copy of the application and submits the required documentation. Then the Central Application Service will process, copy, and distribute the application to each of the programs the candidate specifies. This makes the process easier and uniform. Some programs require that this system be used to apply for a residency (ophthalmology and otolaryngology) and optional for others (neurosurgery and some fellowships). The fee for this service is in addition to other matching fees. Applicants using this service must send all of their application material to the service in one package. The materials to be submitted are the same as those used for the paper or ERAS applications, but unlike these, where staggered accumulation is permissible, for the CAS everything must be submitted at the same time. While there is no true deadline for the submission of this material, the practical target for submission is mid-August. Additional information and answers to frequently asked questions about the CAS are available at its Web site (Figure 15-5).

Central Application Service (CAS)

Do you shriek at the idea of filling out dozens of applications for countless training programs around the nation? Fortunately, there is a solution! The Central Application Service distributes applications to residency and fellowship training programs for you. All you have to do is fill out ONE universal application form, gather ONE copy of each of the appropriate documents, and mail your entire package to CAS. We process, copy, and distribute your applications to each of the programs that you request. Depending on the specialty, CAS may be mandatory or optional. There is an additional fee for this service, but using the CAS service assures that your application is both uniform and complete.

Use of the Central Application Service (CAS) is advantageous to all programs, since it reduces their administrative load. Using CAS is also advantageous to you, the applicant, since you will need only one set of documents and you are in complete control of their assembly.

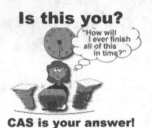

Is this you?

"How will I ever finish all of this in time?"

CAS is your answer!

SF*Match* provides a Central Application Service for the following specialties:

☐ Neurological Surgery Residency Programs
   (CAS is optional for some programs, mandatory for all others)

☐ Neurology Residency Programs NEW!
   (CAS is optional for some programs)

☐ Ophthalmology Residency Programs
   (CAS is mandatory)

☐ Otolaryngology Residency Programs
   (CAS is mandatory)

☐ Head & Neck Oncologic Fellowships
   (CAS is optional for all programs)

Figure 15-4 The San Francisco Web site includes information for candidates about the Central Application Service used by several surgical subspecialties. (Used with permission of the San Francisco Matching Programs.)

CAS Related Pages On This Web Site

▶ **CAS INSTRUCTION MANUAL**

   ☐ Introduction to the CAS Service
   ☐ Step I: Gathering Support Documents
   ☐ Step II: Completing The CAS Application Form
   ☐ Step III: Submitting Your CAS Package
   ☐ Frequently Asked Questions About SF*Match* 's CAS

▶ **DOWNLOADABLE CAS FORMS**

   ☐ FORM: Official CAS Application Forms & Distribution Lists
   ☐ FORM: Returning CAS Documents to the Applicant
   ☐ FORM: Applying to Post-Match Vacancies

Figure 15-5 The San Francisco Matching Programs Web site offers additional information about the Central Application Service they provide. (Used with permission of the San Francisco Matching Programs.)

The Urology Match

Since 1985, the American Urological Association (AUA) has facilitated the matching of students and residency programs in urology. Students interested in a career in urology go through this matching process to obtain their second-year appointment to their specialty residency and go through the regular NRMP for their initial surgical training. The AUA has an excellent general Web site and specific information about their match (Figures 15-6 and 15-7). The AUA charges a $50 fee for the matching service, but this fee is independent of the number of program to which you apply. (Urology training programs are charged $75 for each vacancy listed in the current match.) Like other matches, the results of this match are announced early (late January) so you can use the information to help plan your Rank Order List for the NRMP match to your preliminary surgical program. A general timetable for the urology matching process is shown in Table 15-2.

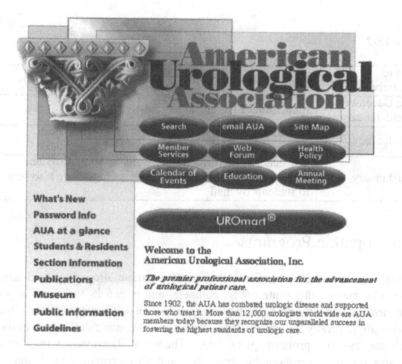

Figure 15-6 The American Urological Association Web site\i provides a large amount of information about the career of urology as well as information about the residency training process and its match. (Used by permission of the American Urological Association.)

AUA Residency Matching Program For Urology

Information for Resident Candidates and Program Directors

INDEX

Registration Form	Violations
Match Schedule	Maximize Your Chances
General Information	Results
Binding Contract	Safeguards
Interviews	Match Overview
Post-Interview Contact	Questions and Answers
Training Requirements	Programs Participating in 2000 Urology Match
Matching Fee	Statistics
Urology Vacancy Hotline	Sample Preference List
Rank-Ordered Preference Lists	Your Suggestions To Us
Program Switching	

Figure 15-7 The American Urological Association Web site has all the information you need to apply for the matching process in urology. (Used by permission of the American Urological Association.)

Table 15-2

June to December	Register with the urology match and apply to programs
Late December to mid-January	Rank Order Lists are submitted
Mid-January	**Deadline** for receipt or Rank Order Lists from both programs and applicants
Mid-January	The match is performed and results faxed to programs and dean's (or student affairs) office; results are also sent to students by mail

Osteopathic Programs

Graduates of osteopathic medical schools often pursue allopathic residencies. Those who choose this route apply, compete, and match in the same way as other medical students, although they compete as independent candidates. These students are generally indistinguishable from their allopathic colleagues in their match success and program placements. There are, however, a number of programs specific to osteopathic graduates, and all osteopathic graduates are strongly suggested to take an American Osteopathic Association (AOA)-approved, one-year osteopathic rotating internship. This internship is intended to provide exposure to a wide range of specialties, giving the future specialist a holistic foundation to his or her subsequent residency training.

All AOA-approved residency training programs require satisfactory completion of an osteopathic internship. Similarly, completion of an AOA-approved internship is required for the osteopathic specialty certification examination. Some states deny licensure to osteopathic physicians unless they have completed an AOA-approved internship. Students who do not participate in the osteopathic match, and choose to take allopathic (non–AOA-approved) first-year graduate training instead of an osteopathic rotating internship, are not assured of receiving AOA approval for their training. Only interns for whom AOA has a signed AOA contract (waiver) may receive credit for this type of internship.

National Matching Services, Inc. (NMS) administers the matching process for osteopathic internships. Registration for this service is recommended to take place in the early fall (usually early September) and costs $80, which is collected on behalf of the AOA. Like some of the surgical specialties discussed above, this is a paper-based matching program with its own set of deadlines (Table 15-3). This match specifically offers a couple's matching option for its participants. The results of the matching process are posted on the NMS Web site at 12:00 noon, eastern standard time, on their match day (late in January). Information for unmatched students is posted at the same time. Consequently, there is no dreaded telephone call or message before match day; everyone finds out together.

The AOA and NMS provide all the information necessary for their matching program on their Web sites (Figure 15-8).

Table 15-3

June	Students register with the NMS and apply to programs
August to September	Programs register with NMS and information about programs is sent to registrants in October
Late September	**Recommended date** for student registration
Late October	Rank Order Lists are distributed
Early January	**Deadline** for receipt of Rank Order Lists from both programs and applicants
Late January	The match is performed and results faxed to programs and dean's (or student affairs) office. Results are also sent to students by mail and available on the Web site
Match +30	Signed contracts must be returned or the student is barred from accepting any AOA-internship for 1 year

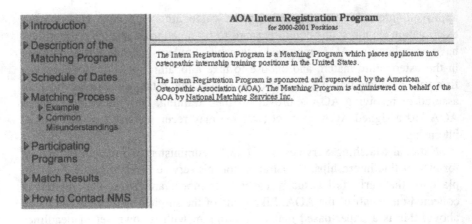

Figure 15-8 The National Matching Service and American Osteopathic Association Web sites have all the information you need to apply for the osteopathic match. (Used by permission of the National Matching Services, Inc.)

Canadian Programs

Residency programs offered in Canada participate in the matching service managed by Canadian Resident Matching Service (CaRMS). The CaRMS compiles a directory of available first year postgraduate programs in Canadian medical schools. Like other matching services, the Canadian Resident Matching Service is a not-for-profit, fee-for-service corporation that works in close cooperation with Canadian medical schools and students. Unlike most other matching programs, the CaRMS handles the application process for its candidates as well. (Some of the specialties matches administered by the San Francisco Match offer such a service as well.)

To keep applicants informed, the CaRMS publishes a newsletter three times during the matching cycle to answer questions about the match and disseminate program updates and changes in schedules and requirements. It also maintain a Web site that contains information about the CaRMS match and detailed information about the residencies that participate (Figure 15-9).

The Canadian Residency Matching Program is somewhat smaller than the United States version, matching 1,149 candidates in 1999. This smaller size, however, allows it to provide a great deal of information directly to its participants. Despite size differences, the match rate for participants in the CaRMS is similar to the NRMP, with 56.8% of students getting their first choice of programs and 78.3% matching to one of their top three picks (in 1999).

CaRMS Program Directory
1999-2000

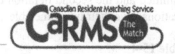

Please read this introduction

The *CaRMS Program Directory* is an up-to-date listing of postgraduate programs available at 13 of the 16 Canadian medical schools. It is revised frequently as programs are updated, requirements change and other new information is sent to CaRMS by the various medical schools across Canada.

Because students applying for postgraduate positions depend on the information listed in the *CaRMS Directory*, beginning in September, changes are announced in the newsletter, *Applying To You*, and highlighted in the program indices with the following symbols:

UPDATED!   **NEW!**

Please also take note of the last date of revision of a program description at the bottom of each program page.

Indices for Programs

 Programs by specialty.

including an option to print mailing labels by specialty

 Programs by university

 Programs offering positions, but not through CaRMS

Figure 15-9 The Canadian Residency Matching Service Web site has complete information about participating Canadian residencies. (Used by permission of the Canadian Residency Matching Service.)

Unlike the U.S. match, the Canadian match is carried out in two iterations: The first is for Canadian applicants, and the second is for unmatched Canadian students and other qualified applicants. If you are not a Canadian citizen or landed immigrant, you may not be eligible for some Canadian positions, so check the details spelled out by the CaRMS on its Web site before you apply for the second iteration match. Canadian students who are unmatched in the first iteration of the CaRMS are automatically (and at no additional cost) entered into a second iteration match. (The signed CaRMS residency match contract from the first iteration binds applicants to their match results in the second iteration of the match.) If a student is unmatched in the first iteration, the student is asked to request new reference letters, write a new personal letter, and be available for telephone interviews in mid- to late March. A second set of Rank Order Lists is submitted and the second iteration of the match carried out. The first and second iterations have their own timetables, as shown in Table 15-4.

Table 15-4

July	Application and registration material are distributed to final-year medical students by undergraduate office; a directory of residency programs is available on-line
September 30	**Deadline** for registration
October 15	Program confirmation lists mailed to students and independent applicants for verification. Preliminary list of applicants mailed to program directors for their information (Changes permitted for 1 week, with late fee)
November 1	**Deadline** for CaRMS to receive dean's letter, medical school transcript, and personal letters
November 15	Applicant files sent from CaRMS to programs by courier
Early January	Rank Order Lists mailed to applicants and programs
February 1	**Deadline** for registration in second iteration for candidates not part of the first iteration
Mid February	Confirmations of ranking mailed to every student and program director whose rank order list is received by this date
Late February	**Deadline** for receipt of Rank Order Lists
Match day –2	Unmatch day; list of positions in the second iteration match will be mailed to second iteration registrants and unmatched applicants from the First Iteration, and will be available at CaRMS
Match day (mid-march)	Match results released and are made available on the Web site
Late March	Rank Order Lists are due for the second iteration (generally about 10 days after Match day)
End of March	Second iteration results announced

Canadian medical graduates are free to participate in the NRMP (though the Canadian government discourages it) and have access to the ERAS system through the CaRMS. The CaRMS levies a charge of $50 (Canadian, plus GST or HST) to access the ERAS system. Canadian students do participate in the NRMP as independent candidates. Students may register with the NRMP concurrently with their registration with CaRMS; however, the Canadian match supersedes the United States NRMP match. These students may remain in the CaRMS match on the understanding that, if they are matched in the first iteration, they will automatically be withdrawn (without notice) from the U.S. match. If students are unmatched in the first iteration, they remain in the U.S. match. If students are matched in NRMP match, they are withdrawn from the second phase of the CaRMS. Canadian students may choose to participate solely in the NRMP if they desire, though because the Canadian match has an earlier announcement date, most students of Canadian medical schools register in both.

CaRMS Handbook 2000 Match

The *CaRMS Handbook*, which is published annually, contains information for students registering for the match. It details eligibility requirements, procedures, statistics on the previous year's match, CaRMS policies, and provides the timetable for the current year.

Addresses of Related Organizations

CaRMS policies

Statistics on the 1999 match

Basis for eligibility for First Iteration and Second Iteration of the Match

- Students graduating from Canadian medical schools
- Students graduating from medical schools in the United States
- Prior year graduates of CACMS/LCME accredited medical schools
- International medical school graduates
  - Frequently Asked Questions
  - Provincial Restrictions
- National Resident Matching Program (NRMP) applicants
- Electronic Application Service to programs in the United States

First iteration of the match

- Timetable for the first iteration of the 2000 Match
- Registering with CaRMS
  - Canadian Medical Students
  - U.S. Medical Students
  - National Defense Funded Students
  - Couples Matching
  - Others
- Registration Documents
  - CaRMS Applicant Match Contract
  - Application for Postgraduate Medical Training
  - Applicant's Designation List
  - Curriculum vitae
  - Fees
  - Late application
  - Deleting application
- Supporting documents
  - Medical school transcript
  - Dean's letter
  - Letters of reference
  - Personal letters

Figure 15-10 The Canadian Residency Matching Service Web site has a complete handbook of information for students interested in Canadian residencies. (Used by permission of the Canadian Residency Matching Service.)

A complete handbook for all aspects of the Canadian Residents Matching Service is available at its Web site (Figure 15-10).

International Graduates

Medical graduates from outside the United States, Canada, or Puerto Rico face slightly different hurdles. Regardless of citizenship, if you did not graduate from an ACGME-accredited medical school in the United States, Canada, or Puerto Rico, you must participate in the NRMP as an independent candidate. There are several different designations for students who are independent candidates (Table 15-5).

Table 15-5

Independent Applicant Categories	Code
Student/graduate of a school of osteopathic medicine	94
U.S. citizen student/graduate of a foreign medical school	95
Student/graduate of a Canadian medical school	96
Non-U.S. citizen student/graduate of a foreign medical school	97
Student/graduate of a Fifth Pathway Program	98
Graduate physician of a U.S. allopathic school not sponsored by a U.S. medical school	99

The NRMP requires that students and graduates of foreign medical schools pass all examinations required for Educational Commission for Foreign Medical Graduates (ECFMG) certification before they can participate in the match. The ECFMG requires that applicants for certification pass the medical science examination in the basic medical and clinical sciences, an English-language proficiency test, and, if necessary, the Clinical Skills Assessment (CSA). The NRMP requires Fifth Pathway Program students and graduates to have passed USMLE Step 1 and Step 2 (or their equivalents). Fifth Pathway Program students and graduates are not required to take an English-language proficiency test or the Clinical Skills Assessment to participate in the match. Information about these requirements is available directly from the ECFMG.

International medical applicants must pay a nonrefundable registration fee of $90 to enroll in the match. This fee must be paid in U.S. dollars, drawn on a U.S. bank, by check or money order; Visa or MasterCard is also acceptable. All other fees for participating in the NRMP are the same for independent candidates and those from U.S. ACGME certified schools. International graduates are bound by the same deadlines and have the same opportunities for such options as advanced programs and the couple's match. The ECFMG acts as the clearinghouse for information and your site for ERAS software. Information about the results of the match is sent to the ECFMG, but most candidates get their results from the NRMP Web site on match day.

The Couple's Match

Couples (or other pairs) who wish to link their matching process can do so through the NRMP couple's match. Matching as a couple can link your program choices together so that they can be matched into a combination of programs suited to your needs. In creating pairs of program choices on their Rank Order Lists, couples have no limitations on how they construct their lists. This allows the members of a couple to remain near each other geographically or express other preferences about the appointments they need or want. Couples can be matched into a combination of programs suited to their personal needs. In creating pairs of programs, you can mix specialties, program types (preliminary or transitional, categorical, and advanced), and geographic locations; the choices are up to you. If you are both in the same specialty, the couple's match can link your residencies so that they occur in the same institution, or can place you in different programs so you don't have to work directly together.

To use the couples match, each partner of the couple enrolls individually in the Match and indicates in the WebROLIC system that he or she wants to be in the Match as part of a couple. The couple will form pairs of choices on their primary Rank Order Lists, which are then considered in rank order in the Match. That is, the couple will match to the most preferred pair of programs on their Rank Order Lists where each partner has been offered a position. Each partner must have the same number of ranks (including "no matches"). Therefore, each program ranked must be paired with an active program or by an indication of "no match" (NRMP program code = 999999) by the other partner. Entering this code indicates that one partner is willing to go unmatched if the other can get a position in the program designated at that rank. Partners listed as a couple are treated by the system solely as a couple. This means that if they do not obtain a match as a couple, the system will not run their lists separately to find a possible match for each individual. This is why couples use the "no match" option so that they are not both in the scramble at the same time.

To understand this process, let's look at a hypothetical couple; Peggy and Bill. For the purposes of this example, we do not need to know what specialty they are pursuing, or even if it is the same, only that they will both be using the NRMP system. Both register for the match in the same way as the rest of their classmates. Both Peggy and Bill have applied to the programs that interest them, have had their interviews, and it is time for them to develop their Rank Order Lists. For the couples match, it is very important that Peggy and Bill go through several preliminary steps to determine the final list they will submit.

To begin with, both partners should sit down and decide what their ideal Rank Order List would look like if they were independent of the other person (Figure 15-11). This is a preliminary list only and helps each person to consolidate his or her thoughts. The lists do not (and most often will not) match in any way. That is allowed at this point.

Peggy	Bill
Washington — City General Chicago — County Los Angeles — Doctor's Boston — Midtown Washington — Metro	Chicago — Western General Chicago — Memorial Tucson — General Chicago — University Washington — Regional Washington — City General

Figure 15-11

Peggy	Bill
Washington — City General	Washington — Regional
Washington — City General	Washington — City General
Chicago — County	Chicago — Western General
Chicago — County	Chicago — Memorial
Chicago — County	Chicago — University
Los Angeles — Doctor's	Chicago — Western General
Los Angeles — Doctor's	Chicago — Memorial
Los Angeles — Doctor's	Chicago — University
Washington — Metro	Washington — Regional
Washington — Metro	Washington — City General
Washington — City General	NO MATCH
Chicago — County	NO MATCH
Los Angeles — Doctor's	NO MATCH
Boston — Midtown	NO MATCH
Washington — Metro	NO MATCH
NO MATCH	Chicago— Western General
NO MATCH	Chicago — Memorial
NO MATCH	Tucson — General
NO MATCH	Chicago — University
NO MATCH	Washington — Regional

Figure 15-12

Next, Peggy and Bill will compare their lists and try to decide what pairings of these options are best (Figure 15-12). These pairing are not ranked in order of preference, just which matching of simultaneous appointment would work and which would not. Couples decide these lists based on factors such as the desirability of programs, competitiveness of the programs, and the competitiveness of each individual of the pair. When one partner is in a particularly competitive field and the other is not, this may slant the level of flexibility the couple may feel for one or the other partner.

The next step for the couple is to take this list of pairings and decide what their preference would be for each of the possible pairings. This list will be used for each partner to enter as his or her Rank Order List (Figure 15-13). When this list is entered, both Peggy and Bill will have to indicate that their list is part of a couple's match and each must indicate the other as the matching list. Note that for each pairing in which one partner would be intentionally left unmatched, the program code "999999" is entered. (In the NMS match for osteopathic graduates the code is "8888".) This signals the system to match one partner but not the other. This reduces the chance of both going unmatched and fulfills the requirement that the Rank Order Lists be the same lengths. (That is, every entry on one list must have a corresponding program or "999999" entry on the other.)

Peggy	Bill
Chicago — County	Chicago — Western General
Chicago — County	Chicago — Memorial
Chicago — County	Chicago — University
Los Angeles — Doctor's	Chicago — Western General
Los Angeles — Doctor's	Chicago — Memorial
Los Angeles — Doctor's	Chicago — University
Washington — City General	Washington — Regional
Washington — City General	Washington — City General
Washington — Metro	Washington — Regional
Washington — Metro	Washington — City General
Washington — City General	999999
999999	Chicago — Western General
999999	Chicago — Memorial
Chicago — County	999999
999999	Tucson — General
Los Angeles — Doctor's	999999
999999	Chicago — University
Boston — Midtown	999999
999999	Washington — Regional
Washington — Metro	999999

Figure 15-13

Once the Rank Order Lists have been entered into the computer and the deadline has passed, the matching process begins. The computer will check each candidate's list to identify those programs that would extend an individual offer (Figure 15-14, indicated by "#"). In our example, Peggy receives offers from Chicago—County, Washington—City General, and Washington - Metro. Bill receives offers from Chicago—Memorial and Washington—Regional. The computer next identifies those pairings in which both Peggy and Bill had offers (boxed pairs). The final step is to choose the highest ranking of these pairs as the match.

	Peggy	Bill	
#	Chicago — County	Chicago — Western General	
#	Chicago — County	Chicago — Memorial	#
#	Chicago — County	Chicago — University	
	Los Angeles — Doctor's	Chicago — Western General	
	Los Angeles — Doctor's	Chicago — Memorial	#
	Los Angeles — Doctor's	Chicago — University	
#	Washington — City General	Washington — Regional	#
#	Washington — City General	Washington — City General	
#	Washington — Metro	Washington — Regional	#
#	Washington — Metro	Washington — City General	
#	Washington — City General	999999	
	999999	Chicago — Western General	
	999999	Chicago — Memorial	#
	Chicago — County	999999	
	999999	Tucson — General	
	Los Angeles — Doctor's	999999	
	999999	Chicago — University	
	Boston — Midtown	999999	
	999999	Washington — Regional	#
#	Washington — Metro	999999	

Figure 15-14

Had the Chicago programs not extended offers to one or both Peggy and Bill, the next match on their list (Washington—City General and Washington—Regional) would have been chosen. If Peggy had received only her Washington offers and Bill had received only an offer from Tucson, they would have ended up with Peggy assigned to Washington—City General and Bill left to scramble for a position outside the match. If the couple had not included these "no match" options, they would have remained unmatched because the matching system will not treat them as individuals if they cannot be matched as a pair.[1]

Just like with individual Rank Order Lists, the ranking should reflect the individual's (and the couple's combined) true feelings about desirability and should not be driven by the chances of a match. Similarly, neither partner should list a program that he or she would not be happy to receive as a match. Because of the intricacies of attempting to pair two candidates at the same time, it is wise to list all acceptable programs to reduce the chances of being unmatched completely.

---

[1] This is a very simplified version of the matching process that does not take into account the dynamic nature of each offer by a program. The availability of a tentative match is based on the same principles discussed in Chapter 16

The cost of the couple's match is calculated in a slightly different manner from that of the single candidate. In the couple's match, there is a $15 per person fee to be a part of the couple's process. This fee covers registration and up to fifteen unique programs and up to 300 entries on the person's Rank Order List. Additional programs cost $30 each and each rank listing cost $15 each. Each partner in a pair may have different fees based on this system, but the system does take into account the longer Rank Order List caused by combinations and permutations of paired programs.

Some special circumstances are worth mentioning. If a partner's rank is for an advanced position, a Supplemental Rank Order List for that program must also be prepared by that partner unless the required first-year program has already been completed. If both partners choose an advanced position, each must prepare separate Supplemental Rank Order Lists. The choices made should be geographically acceptable to both partners. If both partners match to advanced programs, their Supplemental Rank Order Lists are not treated as a unit (pair) in the match, so that the normal processes of keeping the preferences matched up do not apply. You should also note that if one partner withdraws from the match, the other partner's Rank Order List will remain in the system and will be used in the match as for a single candidate. The withdrawal of one does not affect the other.

What happens when one partner is part of the NRMP and the other is part of a specialty match? The couples system is not engineered to handle this situation and you are somewhat on your own. While you can both try to juggle your Rank Order Lists and hope for the best, this is somewhat risky. Unless you are going to a large metropolitan area (with lots of programs and slots), using this approach will generally leave one partner or the other with a very short rank list, placing that person at risk for being unmatched. This situation may be preferable to being placed at programs that are widely separated. Another option is for the partner in the less competitive field to expand his or her list through the inclusion of transitional or preliminary positions in addition to the preferred specialty. This might mean ending up with a couple that both matches and are geographically close, but with one partner forced into a "holding pattern" for a year while awaiting a specialty opening in the preferred location.

Only you can decide the best options for yourselves, and each couple may be different in its solution. Discuss this openly with your advisors and with those you meet when you interview. If one or both partners are particularly desirable, a program might consider offering positions outside of the match and reducing their match quota by an appropriate amount. Don't get your hopes up; this doesn't happen very often and it's against the rules.

Shared Positions

The ultimate couple's match is the shared position. Very few programs offer shared-residency positions (Figure 15-15). In a shared residency, two individuals share one position, usually alternating months or rotations on clinical services, with time off to devote to families, research, or other pursuits. The time it takes for each person to complete the residency training is generally doubled. To apply for a shared position, each of the applicants enrolls individually in the match and then together they submit a Shared Residency Pair Form. These applicants cannot apply as individuals for full-time positions in the match. The two applicants are assigned a single NRMP applicant code and will be included in the NRMP Applicant Listing as a combined name. The shared pair submits only one Rank Order List. As with all lists, this should include all of the acceptable shared positions that both applicants agree to be matched to. If the pair is matched to a full-time position, both individuals are bound to accept it, so list only positions you both agree upon. If one partner of the pair withdraws from the match, the remaining partner must decide on continuing to participate in the match. In this case, a new NRMP code will be assigned to the remaining applicant.

FAMILY PRACTICE

Hospital Name	City	State	Code
U ARKANSAS MED SC-FAYETTEVILLE	FAYETTEVILLE	AR	300220
U ROCHESTER/STRONG MEMORIAL	ROCHESTER	NY	151120
ST JOSEPHS HOSPITAL HEALTH CTR	SYRACUSE	NY	151820

INTERNAL MED CATEGORICAL

Hospital Name	City	State	Code
SALEM HOSPITAL	SALEM	MA	128416
ALBERT EINSTEIN MEDICAL CENTER	PHILADELPHIA	PA	163116

PEDIATRICS

Hospital Name	City	State	Code
UNIV OF MARYLAND MEDICAL CTR	BALTIMORE	MD	125228

Figure 15-15 Only a very few programs offer the option of shared positions. (From National Residency Matching Program, used with permission.)

Special Needs

A small number of students have a disability. The Americans with Disabilities Act (ADA) of 1990 defines "disability" as a physical or mental impairment that substantially limits one or more major life functions. Students with disabilities are often concerned about their ability to compete on an equal basis with their colleagues. It should be apparent that if you have been able to get to the point of applying for residency, you have the drive, stamina, and abilities required to successfully compete for almost any program. The ADA requires that an employer make "reasonable accommodations" for disabled applicants and employees. Since you are applying for a position in a health care field, most physical barriers will have already been addressed by the institution. All that remains will be those specific to your performance as a resident. As long as any accommodations required do not pose an "undue hardship" to the "business operation," the ADA requires that your needs be met.

It is illegal to discriminate on the basis of disability (among other things). Because of the ADA, it is also illegal to ask about the extent of your disability. It is legal to ask about, or even test, your ability to perform the job for which your are applying. For example, it is not legal to ask how well you can see. It is legal to say that you are required to be able to interpret EKGs, x-rays, ultrasonography, or fetal heart rate tracings, and ask if you can perform those tasks. The general question is out of bounds, the specific job-related question is allowed.

It is completely legal, and not a bad idea, for you to volunteer some assessment of your abilities, problems you have faced, and how you have overcome them. This gives you the upper hand in preempting any concerns about your ability to get the job done. If you need special considerations for your interview, let the program know well in advance so they can make the necessary accommodations. You should not hide either your abilities or disabilities. Your disabilities should not be a source of embarrassment or stigma; they are just a part of who you are.

Chapter 16

The Computer Match Process

Each year, the majority of senior students, and many others, participate in the matching process offered by the National Resident matching Program (NRMP). This is the computerized and confidential system of ranking and matching residents and residencies first introduced in 1952. Those are the dry facts. The practical description of the match is that it is a system that can hook up candidates and residencies in such a way that neither party has control, but both receive the most desirable outcome possible. In the case of a tie, the student's wishes are given preference. That said, it is still important that you have some sense of exactly what happens in the month between the time that you file your Rank Order List and the greatly anticipated "match day."

Who Participates?

With the exception of some specialty programs that run their own version of the NRMP match, all residencies and residency candidates take part. Technically, each program and student decides to participate individually. Practically, there is little reason for either a program or student not to participate because it would leave you on the outside looking in. Yes, you could directly negotiate with a program that participates in the match and conclude your own deal, with the program then reducing by one the number of candidates it accepts from the match. Without a major endowment from your family or some extraordinary force of nature to recommend your candidacy, this won't happen.

To participate in the National Residency Matching Program, you must be either a sponsored or an independent applicant (Table 16-1). Independent candidates must submit extra documentation and the NRMP will check the credentials of all independent candidates. (See Chapter 15 for further information.) Residency programs that are accredited by the Accreditation Council for Graduate Medical Education (ACGME) are eligible to offer positions through the NRMP match.

Table 16-1 Categories of NRMP Applicants

Sponsored applicants
- Students enrolled in a medical school accredited by the Liaison Committee on Medical Education (LCME) and certified by their dean as eligible
- Previous graduates from an LCME accredited school and sponsored by a medical school

Independent applicants
- Physicians who graduated from an LCME accredited school but who are not sponsored by a medical school
- Applicants enrolled in or who have graduated from a medical school accredited by the Committee on Accreditation of Canadian Medical Schools
- Applicants enrolled in or who have graduated from a medical school accredited by the American Osteopathic Association
- Applicants enrolled in or who have graduated from a schools not accredited by the LCME
- Applicants enrolled or graduated from Fifth Pathway Programs at a medical school accredited by the LCME

If you are pursuing a career in neurology, neurosurgery, ophthalmology, otolaryngology, or urology, you will participate in your own specialty matching process. Because these are advanced programs, you will still use the NRMP system for your preliminary position. Students who have taken time off between their graduation and residency or are seeking changing specialty tracts will also compete for their positions through the matching process, unless you are pursuing one of the five specialties named above. While the success rate for graduates of school outside of North America seeking positions through the match is lower than that for U.S. graduates, this is the only practical way for these students to find residency slots.

What Does the Match Do?

In the simplest terms, the match takes the rank order lists of all involved candidates and programs and proceeds to shuffle them about until every candidate has an appointment or no other acceptable positions exist. This daunting task actually takes only minutes to complete using extensively tested computer algorithms. These algorithms have come under scrutiny in the past few years to ensure that they accomplish their task with the greatest level of equity for all involved.

To understand how this computer matching takes place, and therefore how to best exploit its power, let us consider a hypothetical match between eight students and four hospitals. Our students and hospitals (Table 16-2) are a cross section of abilities and attitudes, competitiveness and desirability that should be representative.

Table 16-2

Student	Characteristics	Hospital	Characteristics
N.T. Bright	Gullible	Pooh-Pooh U.	Self-absorbed
Esther Confident	Bright, uninformed	County General	Inner city
Valerie Dictorian	Brilliant	Metro Regional	Medium size
Stellar Student	Savvy	Doctor's Hospital	Smaller hospital
Tim Id	Hesitant		
Dee Solid	Well qualified		
Avery Ridge	Middle of the class		
Norm Alson	Great personality		

Table 16-3

Student	1st Choice	2nd Choice	3rd Choice	4th Choice
N.T. Bright	County General	-	-	-
E. Confident	County General	Pooh-Pooh U.	-	-
V. Dictorian	County General	Pooh-Pooh U.	-	-
D. Solid	Pooh-Pooh U.	County General	Metro Regional	Doctor's Hospital
A. Ridge	County General	Pooh-Pooh U.	Doctor's Hospital	Metro Regional
S. Student	County General	Metro Regional	Pooh-Pooh U.	Doctor's Hospital
N. Alson	County General	Pooh-Pooh U.	Metro Regional	Doctor's Hospital
T. Id	Doctor's Hospital	County General	Pooh-Pooh U.	-

(Arranged by NRMP code number)

Each of our students has applied to all four of the hospital programs. Interviews have been granted to all of our sample applicants and the respective players have now made their Rank Order Lists (Table 16-3).

Our first student, Bright, has listed only County General because she believes that the program at County General is going to rank her as their top candidate. While she should be a competitive candidate at other programs, she has chosen to rank only the one program. This is not a good use of the matching system and potentially leaves her vulnerable to the reliability of the information she has about the residency's ranking. As noted in Chapter 14, this information should never be trusted.

Our second student, Esther Confident, is a desirable candidate who is expected to graduate at the very top of her class. She has ranked only two programs. While she believes herself to be a desirable and competitive candidate, her interviews did not go well and she has no guarantee of matching at these programs. By ranking only two hospitals and not listing some "safe" options, she places herself at risk for not matching.

The future Doctor Dictorian has also only ranked two hospitals although she interviewed with all four. She prefers the program at County General and has ranked it first although she is fairly certain that the program at Old Pooh-Pooh U. will be ranking her first. She is using the match well by listing her true preference, rather than trying to ensure she gets her first choice by going with what she believes to be a "sure thing." Since she feels that there is virtually no chance that she will be unmatched (because of P-PU.'s statements), she has not chosen to apply to any less desirable options. As long as her information is reliable, this is a reasonable strategy.

Our friend, Stellar Student, enjoyed her rotation at Doctor's Hospital as a junior student and would be happy to go there for her residency. While she believes that they will rank her highly, she would prefer the other programs. Even though she did not think her interview went well at the other hospitals, she ranks them above Doctor's Hospital. This strategy maximizes the benefit of the matching algorithm, giving her the best chance of both matching and receiving the most desirable appointment from those available to her.

Like Stellar, Mr. Id is reasonably sure that the selection committee at Doctor's Hospital liked him and should rank him highly, and he too would prefer other programs as a final destination. Rather than setting his ranking based on the desirability of each, he has chosen to rank Doctor's first to ensure a match, with the other acceptable programs then listed in order of preference. (He was mugged in the parking lot when he went for his interview at Metro General and has chosen not to rank them for this reason.) This may ensure that he will match somewhere, but the computer has no way of knowing that there is a difference between the ranking supplied and the true wishes of the student. This tactic may result in students avoiding the scramble only to leave them disappointed with their final residency.

Our remaining students, Solid, Ridge, and Alson, are good candidates with acceptable grades from a good-quality medical school. These students interviewed well and have a good chance of matching, although this is not assured. They have each ranked the programs according to their own internal sense of value and desire, even though the results differ from student to student. These students are using the match system to their advantage.

Once the deadline for changes has passed, the Rank Order Lists for candidates and programs are frozen and the program's rankings are shown in Table 16-4.

Table 16-4

Old Pooh-Pooh U	County General	Metro Regional	Doctor's Hospital
V. Dictorian	N. Alson	E. Confident	E. Confident
N. Alson	T. Id	A. Ridge	A. Ridge
	A. Ridge	T. Id	N. Bright
	N. Bright	N. Bright	V. Dictorian
	E. Confident	V. Dictorian	T. Id
	V. Dictorian	D. Solid	S. Student
	D. Solid	N. Alson	D. Solid
	S. Student		N. Alson

Each hospital has two residency positions available. The program director at Old Pooh-Pooh University has always bragged that his program has never had to go very far down their list to fill their slots. Although they interviewed all eight students and a number of other students would be acceptable, he has chosen to rank only their top two choices. The selection committee at Metro Regional Hospital was happy with all but one of the candidates who they met, and they have ranked all of the students with this one exception. The program director at Doctor's Hospital knows that, as a smaller hospital, they are not as competitive as some of their better-known competitors. She feels that she has a good chance of matching with Mr. Id and Ms. Student who both enjoyed their rotations during their junior year. Despite this possibility, the program director has correctly ranked the students based on their perceived desirability, not on the basis of making a match.

Given these Rank Order Lists, what will happen when the computer match process proceeds? Since the computer algorithm is driven by an effort to maximize the outcome for the student, the process begins with the student's list (Table 16-5).

Table 16-5

	Old Pooh-Pooh U.	County General	Metro Regional	Doctor's Hospital
N. Bright	V. Dictorian	N. Alson	E. Confident	E. Confident
County General	N. Alson	T. Id	A. Ridge	A. Ridge
		A. Ridge	T. Id	N. Bright
		N. Bright	N. Bright	V. Dictorian
		E. Confident	V. Dictorian	T. Id
		V. Dictorian	D. Solid	S. Student
		D. Solid	N. Alson	D. Solid
		S. Student		N. Alson

The first student (based, in this case, on the NRMP candidate number) is Ms. Bright. The first (and only) program on her list is County General. The computer checks the Rank Order List from County General and finds that the program still has two positions unfilled (all of their allotted spots) and Ms. Bright is on their list of acceptable candidates. The computer establishes a tentative match and reduces the number of open positions available at County General by one. The computer then moves on to the second student, Esther Confident (Table 16-6).

Table 16-6

	Old Pooh-Pooh U.	County General	Metro Regional	Doctor's Hospital
E. Confident	V. Dictorian	N. Alson	E. Confident	E. Confident
County General	N. Alson	T. Id	A. Ridge	A. Ridge
Old Pooh-Pooh U.		A. Ridge	T. Id	N. Bright
		N. Bright	N. Bright	V. Dictorian
		E. Confident	V. Dictorian	T. Id
		V. Dictorian	D. Solid	S. Student
		D. Solid	N. Alson	D. Solid
		S. Student		N. Alson

The Rank Order List filed by Ms. Confident lists County General first and Old Pooh-Pooh University second, with no other programs listed. The computer checks the list for County General and finds that there is still one unfilled position. In addition, Ms. Confident is on the list of acceptable students. Again a tentative match is established, but now County General is listed as filled. From now on, for any student to be tentatively matched to County General, they must be listed on the hospital's list in a position above that of students Bright and Confident. The computer moves on as the next student's list is retrieved (Table 16-7).

Table 16-7

	Old Pooh-Pooh U.	County General	Metro Regional	Doctor's Hospital
V. Dictorian	V. Dictorian	N. Alson	E. Confident	E. Confident
County General	N. Alson	T. Id	A. Ridge	A. Ridge
Old Pooh-Pooh U		A. Ridge	T. Id	N. Bright
		N. Bright	N. Bright	V. Dictorian
		E. Confident	V. Dictorian	T. Id
		V. Dictorian	D. Solid	S. Student
		D. Solid	N. Alson	D. Solid
		S. Student		N. Alson

Ms. Dictorian's list matches that of Ms. Confident, but this time the results are different. When the computer checks the list for County General, it finds that candidates ranked higher by the hospital already fill all of the residency positions. Consequently, the computer checks the next hospital on the student's list. Old Pooh-Pooh University has an unfilled position and she is on the list, so a tentative match is made, the number of positions available is reduced, and the computer moves on to the list filed by Dee Solid (Table 16-8).

Table 16-8

	Old Pooh-Pooh U.	County General	Metro Regional	Doctor's Hospital
D. Solid	[V. Dictorian]	N. Alson	E. Confident	E. Confident
	N. Alson	T. Id	A. Ridge	A. Ridge
Pooh-Pooh U.		A. Ridge	T. Id	N. Bright
County General		[N. Bright]	N. Bright	V. Dictorian
Metro Regional		[E. Confident]	V. Dictorian	T. Id
Doctor's Hospital		V. Dictorian	[D. Solid]	S. Student
		D. Solid	N. Alson	D. Solid
		S. Student		N. Alson

Ms. Solid's match, like that of Valerie Dictorian's, requires several steps before success is achieved. In the first step, the computer checks the candidate list for Old Pooh-Pooh University and finds that Dee is not listed. The computer checks the next program on the list and finds that is it filled by students ranked higher by the program director at County General. The third program on the list, Metro General has two unfilled positions and Ms. Solid is listed as an acceptable candidate, so a tentative match is established and the appropriate additional changes are made.

Matching the next student on the list, Ridge, illustrates why the matches made so far are only temporary. When the computer attempts to match Ridge to a program, it results in displacing the temporary match made earlier for Ms. Confident (Table 16-9).

Table 16-9

	Old Pooh-Pooh U.	County General	Metro Regional	Doctor's Hospital
A. Ridge	[V. Dictorian]	N. Alson	E. Confident	E. Confident
	N. Alson	T. Id	A. Ridge	A. Ridge
County General		[A. Ridge]	T. Id	N. Bright
Pooh-Pooh U.		[N. Bright]	N. Bright	V. Dictorian
Doctor's Hospital		[E. Confident]	V. Dictorian	T. Id
Metro Regional		V. Dictorian	[D. Solid]	S. Student
		D. Solid	N. Alson	D. Solid
E. Confident		S. Student		N. Alson
County General				
Old Pooh-Pooh U.				

[**Unmatched**]

The computer looks at the list submitted by Avery Ridge and finds that while County General's positions have been filled, Avery is considered to be a more desirable candidate. Therefore, the tentative match with the lowest priority, that of Esther Confident, is broken and a tentative match with Ridge made. The computer now must go back to the programs remaining on Ms. Confident's list.

The sole remaining program on the list did not list that candidate as being acceptable and so Ms. Confident becomes unmatched and will have to try to find her own program through the scramble.

The match for Stellar Student is less disruptive but still requires several steps (Table 16-10).

Table 16-10

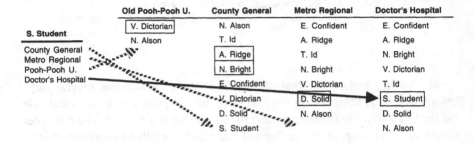

	Old Pooh-Pooh U.	County General	Metro Regional	Doctor's Hospital
S. Student	V. Dictorian	N. Alson	E. Confident	E. Confident
	N. Alson	T. Id	A. Ridge	A. Ridge
County General		A. Ridge	T. Id	N. Bright
Metro Regional		N. Bright	N. Bright	V. Dictorian
Pooh-Pooh U.		E. Confident	V. Dictorian	T. Id
Doctor's Hospital		V. Dictorian	D. Solid	S. Student
		D. Solid	N. Alson	D. Solid
		S. Student		N. Alson

As with some of the previous students, the first attempt to match a program finds the program filled with more preferred students. The second and third hospitals did not rank Stellar, so the computer checks the final entry, that of Doctor's Hospital. Doctor's Hospital still has two unfilled positions and, while not the program director's first choice, Stella was still a very acceptable candidate, and a match is made.

As increasing numbers of tentative matches are made, the chances that a conflict will occur also increase. That is what happens with our next candidate, Norm Alson (Table 16-11).

As we saw with the match of Mr. Ridge, when a program is filled but the candidate is ranked higher on the program's list, the less desirable student is displaced and replaced by the higher-ranking person. In this case, Ms. Bright becomes unmatched although she would have been a tentative match at the Metro Regional or Doctor's Hospital programs. Here the failure to match was not a reflection of the candidate's desirability, but was a function of poor planning and use of the matching system.

Table 16-11

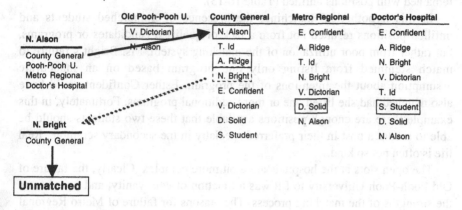

	Old Pooh-Pooh U.	County General	Metro Regional	Doctor's Hospital
N. Alson	V. Dictorian	N. Alson	E. Confident	E. Confident
County General	N. Alson	T. Id	A. Ridge	A. Ridge
Pooh-Pooh U.		A. Ridge	T. Id	N. Bright
Metro Regional		N. Bright	N. Bright	V. Dictorian
Doctor's Hospital		E. Confident	V. Dictorian	T. Id
		V. Dictorian	D. Solid	S. Student
N. Bright		D. Solid	N. Alson	D. Solid
County General		S. Student		N. Alson

Unmatched

Table 16-12

	Old Pooh-Pooh U.	County General	Metro Regional	Doctor's Hospital
T. Id	V. Dictorian	N. Alson	E. Confident	E. Confident
Doctor's Hospital	N. Alson	T. Id	A. Ridge	A. Ridge
County General		A. Ridge	T. Id	N. Bright
Pooh-Pooh U.		N. Bright	N. Bright	V. Dictorian
		E. Confident	V. Dictorian	T. Id
		V. Dictorian	D. Solid	S. Student
		D. Solid	N. Alson	D. Solid
		S. Student		N. Alson

Table 16-13

	Old Pooh-Pooh U.	County General	Metro Regional	Doctor's Hospital
Unmatched	V. Dictorian	N. Alson	D. Solid	T. Id
N. Bright		A. Ridge		S. Student
E. Confident				

Our last student, Id is an easy match (Tble 16-12) although he could have matched at his more desirable program (County General) had he listed his programs according to his true wishes.

At this point all students have been matched to a program that will accept them and this match has been made with the program ranked highest on the student's list. In no case are there any acceptable pairings that result in both the applicant and the program improving its position. (In technical parlance, this is called a stable match.) The only students remaining are unmatched because no program with unfilled positions ranked the student. Once these conditions have been met, the matches are considered "final" and the match closes. The result is that of our eight students, two remained unmatched while three got their first choice and one each received their second, third and fourth picks. Two hospitals remained with positions unfilled (Table 16-13).

In this hypothetical matching, the presence of unmatched students and unfilled positions resulted not from a lack of qualified candidates or programs, but rather from poor utilization of the matching system. Ms. Bright's failure to match stemmed from listing only one program based on an inaccurate assumption about the intentions of the program. Esther Confident could have also matched had she listed one or more additional programs. Fortunately, in this example there are enough positions available that these two students should be able to secure a post in their preferred specialty in the secondary scramble. Real life is often not so kind.

The open slots at the hospitals are a bit more complex. Clearly, the failure of Old Pooh-Pooh University to fill was a function of ego, vanity, and poor use of the strengths of the matching process. The reasons for failure of Metro Regional to fill its positions are less apparent. It correctly listed only those students whom it would be willing to accept as residents. Because the system is driven by the students' wishes, it failed to fill because students preferred other programs. Though Dee Solid was not among Metro's first choices, she was an acceptable candidate. In a similar way, Metro was not Dee's first preference, but it too was an acceptable option. In the end, both Metro and Dee should be happy with their coming association.

Who Wins?

The winners in the matching process are those who use the system wisely. The bias toward the students' ranking gives them the edge, but the effect is minimal. In a study reported in 1997, Roth and Peranson found that the difference between a student-driven match and a program-driven one affected less than 0.1% of all applicants. In the five years studied, the student-driven system resulted in only one additional unmatched applicant being matched, while another lost his matchup, resulting in no net gain.

In a stable, "applicant proposing" (student-driven) match, there is little the student can do to improve the match by using a Rank Order List that differs from his or her true preference. As we saw in our hypothetical example, there is no advantage, and a potential disadvantage, in submitting anything other than an honest reflection of your fancy. Like true love, you may not be able to explain to anyone else how you arrived at your list, but you don't have to.

One question that might be posed would be whether there is a preference for those students who the computer first considers and matches. The answer is no. It turns out that in a stable match no matter what order of student lists is used, the same students will remain unmatched and the same programs will stay unfilled. There is no advantage in trying to get a lower number or changing your last name to Abbington. It won't have any effect.

Chapter 17

Match Day

Your quest is almost over. By the time match day approaches in March, the process is out of your control. For good or ill, once the deadline for finalizing your Rank Order List has past, the die has been cast. All that remains is to find out the results. That is what match day is all about.

That simple description of fact belies the impact that everyone involved feels. Whether you are a student, family member, program director, chairman, or dean, this day stands out like no other. It is a mixture of apprehension and relief, the joy of seeing a new phase of your life unfold and the bittersweet passing of another season.

What Happens?

While the focus of match day is the announcement of the matching results, the events of match day actually cover a four-day period:

- Match day minus three (Monday)—At 12:00 noon eastern standard time (EST) the NRMP posts a list of matched and unmatched candidates on its Internet site. This same information is also made available through the NRMP dial-in telephone system. (Have your candidate number and PIN ready.) The dean's office, office of student affairs, or other appropriate officials at your school will also receive information about any of their candidates who have been unmatched. Many students eagerly check one of these sources to find out if they will be a part of the scramble for unfilled positions, or can relax and wait for Match day when the results will be announced. For those too timid to check for themselves, the dean's office will, in most cases, try to track down any students who are unmatched. Whether you choose to check for yourself, or want to wait for the telephone *not* to ring, you should plan to be accessible during this time. Independent candidates can contact the dean's office at their sponsoring school. Foreign medical graduates should contact the offices of the ECFMG. For the few students who are unmatched, you will have to wait twenty-four hours to find out what positions are still open.

- Match day minus two (Tuesday)—At 11:30 am EST, the NRMP posts a list of filled and unfilled programs on its Web site. This list is available to the programs immediately, but only becomes available to applicants at 12:00 noon (EST) on that day. It is against NRMP rules for unmatched applicants to contact programs before this time even though there is a half-hour advanced window in which the programs know they are unfilled. After 12:00 Noon (EST) unmatched students can find out what their options are and begin the process of "scrambling" for a position.

- Match day (Thursday)—The dry facts are that the results are posted to the NRMP Web site and may be viewed after 1:00 pm EST. If you are an independent candidate or a foreign medical graduate applying through the ECFMG, this will be how you find out the name of your residency. For most U.S. students, the process involves more ceremony. The distribution of the results can vary from stopping by the dean's office to pick up an envelope, to a major convocation complete with families, friends, speeches, and bands. Some schools allow students to open their envelopes as soon as they get them, others ask all the candidates to hold the envelopes until everyone has received theirs and a signal is given. This is a big event in everyone's life. It is even common for local television stations to provide camera coverage for inclusion in the evening news broadcast. Although each program knows who it will be getting from the match before the candidates find out their destinations, it is against NRMP policy for the program to make any contact with students before the announcement is officially made.

Getting Set

Unless you have no option, you should be on the campus of your medical school during the week of match day, in case you need access to, or advice from, your advisor. The announcement of the match results is also a rite of passage that should not be missed and is best shared with your classmates and family. Most schools allow senior students to have match day off from other obligations, but you may want to arrange beforehand to have some time protected just in case you need time to be on the telephone. If you don't need the time (and we hope you don't), you can continue your clinical duties. It is better to have made arrangements in advance than to do it at the last minute.

Personal Preparations

Besides making tentative plans for the celebratory dinner, party, or telephone calls, you need to do some mental preparation for the days before match day. While everyone hopes that he or she will match, and the majority of U.S. students do, give some brief thought to your plan B. How would you react if you don't match? What options do you see? Do you know the resources available to assist you? Where will your advisors be if you need them? Do you have the telephone number of the dean's office in case of emergency? While these preparations will not lessen the tumult of finding yourself among the unmatched, it will provide some cushioning at a time when your thinking may not be the clearest.

Once the "unmatch day" passes, be sure you know your school's plans for distributing the results. Nothing says you have to participate—you could, after all, just go to the Web site—but there is almost no reason not to be a part of the excitement. Even if you think you are going to be disappointed with the results, or worse have found out you are unmatched, be there with your head held high. No one will ever know. This is your public persona.

Public Persona

As a part of the rules governing the NRMP match, both you and the program you are matched with have agreed to carry through with the residency position. The program is obligated to offer you the spot and you are obligated to accept it. As we have said repeatedly, this means that if you put a program on your list and the program has put you on its list, you both have tacitly agreed that you would be happy with the outcome. Consequently, there is no reason for the world to see anything but a big smile when you open the envelope. (Don't worry, if you are unmatched there is generally an envelope for you just like everyone else and you should have the advantage of already knowing where you are going, thanks to the scramble—the laugh is on them.)

Because your Rank Order List is completely confidential, absolutely no one can know your final ranking unless you tell them. The dean may announce with pride the percentage of your school's students that got their first choice, etc., but no one need ever know if you did not get your first choice. On match day, everyone can, and should be, a winner.

The Scramble

Every year, about a thousand United States graduates (about 6% of U.S. applicants) will end up with without an assignment on match day. It doesn't mean you are a bad person, you are too dumb to be a doctor, or that you need to change deodorants. This most often happens because of a poorly constructed

Rank Order List, ranking too few programs, or applying to a very competitive specialty without a backup preliminary or transitional option. Hang in there, all is not lost.

What should you do if you get the dreaded call from the dean's office? First, don't panic. You should also delay the gnashing of teeth, chest beating, and hair pulling; save that for your residency. You will want to move quickly to appraise your options. Meet with the designated staff in the dean's office, the program director at your institution, the department chairman, your advisor, and your mentor. Contact them immediately and meet with them soon after. If you can't find your first choice, move down the list until you get help from someone. Since at this point you will not know (and can't find out) what programs have unfilled portions, the purpose of this meeting is to evaluate your battle plan for the next day.

Your attack begins with deciding if you are going to stay with your choice of specialty, consider a different, but related, specialty, or pursue a transitional option. The decision among these options is a personal one and will be driven by many factors including the competitiveness of your original choice, your geographic portability, and your vision of your future. A mentor, advisor, family member, or spouse can often provide the outside perspective needed to help with the decision. Even if you have already considered these factors and arrived at a resolution for these concerns, you will want someone in the school to be available to assist with the mechanics of the scramble. If you have a choice, pick someone knowledgeable with training in the field to help look at the programs open to you. Make an appointment for the next day at noon to look at the list of open positions.

While your are waiting for the unmatched positions list to be posted, gather up the papers you will need for the next day. You will want to go to the dean's office and get a copy of your transcript. If you can get a copy of the dean's letter, do that as well. (If the office will not give these directly to you, find out whom to contact the next day in case you have to have the letter and transcript faxed to any prospective program.) You will want a clean copy of your application form or a printout of your ERAS application. A copy of your CV and personal statement round out the material you may need to fax as part of an emergency application.

On match day minus two, you and your battle team should meet around an Internet-connected computer and download the list of open positions in the field or fields your seek. Quickly make a working list. If any of the programs that have openings were on your initial list, or better yet you applied to but did not interview, go for these first. If your advisor has some acquaintance with the program, have him or her get on the telephone and call right then on your behalf; otherwise, get on the telephone yourself. Ask to speak to the program director or his or her designee. Explain your situation and interest in the unfilled position. The director will understand—he or she is just as traumatized by not matching as you are. Offer to fax any information the director may need and do so immediately.

Negotiate aggressively. Both you and the program want to have this situation resolved as quickly as possible. Ask how soon you may have a decision. Leave multiple telephone numbers where you can be reached. Offer to call back, and do so. Stay on top of things.

While you are waiting for the program to call back, don't sit idly. Pick up the telephone and contact the next program on your list. (Don't tie up the only telephone line if you expect a call back.) If all the programs would be equally acceptable, go through the same process with program numbers two or three. If an offer comes through, take it, but then quickly notify the other programs you have contacted to withdraw you application. This allows the slower programs to offer the position to some other equally nervous student.

If a program asks for an interview, either withdraw your application or insist that it be handled by telephone in the next few hours. You cannot afford to lose the time involved, opening yourself up to the loss of a residency of any type. All programs should understand this and have an equal stake in resolving their own situation quickly. Any program director who does not seem to understand this is not a director you want to work for; run away.

Once you have accepted an offer, ask for a confirmation of the offer by fax, with a hard copy sent to you by express mail or courier. Without some form of documentation, do not consider your search concluded. Offer to send the program clean copies of any of the materials you have faxed, so that it can include them in its files.

When the dust settles, be sure to thank the people involved who helped to pull the fat out of the fire. While this is why we do our job, it is still nice to be appreciated. It does not have to be fancy; a heartfelt smile and thank you make it all worthwhile. Remember we are proud of you, and like to see you succeed as well.

Above all, remember that good candidates and good programs often end up disconnected in the match process. Even if you go through the scramble, you can still chase your dreams, finally proving that you are, indeed, anybody's match.

Chapter 18
Resources and References

Resources for Further Information

The references listed below should be consulted by prospective graduate medical students before choosing a graduate medical program:

COTH Directory/Educational Programs and Services
This publication lists the particular residency programs that are offered by all U.S. teaching hospitals belonging to the Council of Teaching Hospitals (COTH) as well as the accredited U.S. medical schools with which they are affiliated.

COTH Survey of Housestaff Stipends, Benefits, and Funding
This annual publication reports data on stipends, health and nonhealth benefits, teaching hospital expenditures, and sources of funding for house staff stipends and benefits. It also includes nationwide mean and median stipend data aggregated by region and hospital ownership.

Academic Medicine
The official journal of the AAMC, *Academic Medicine* may contain articles on curricular innovations and opportunities in graduate medical education.

Each of these publications is available at most medical and undergraduate college libraries. Individual copies or subscriptions may be purchased by writing to the following address:

Association of American Medical Colleges
ATTN: Membership and Publication Orders
2450 N Street, NW
Suite 340
Washington, DC 20037-1411
(202) 828-0416
(202) 828-1125 fax
http://www.aamc.org

The American Medical Association (AMA) has additional information which should be reviewed:

Graduate Medical Education Directory
This publication lists the Accreditation Council on Graduate Medical Education (ACGME) approved residency programs in the United States for the twenty-four recognized specialties in medicine. The directory (also known as "The Green Book") is available at most medical and undergraduate college libraries or may be purchased through the AMA.

Fellowship and Residency Electronic Interactive Database Access System (AMA-FRIEDA)
FREIDA is a database that provides general information on all ACGME-accredited graduate medical education programs. The system may be accessed from the American Medical Association's home page, or directly at:

http://www.ama-assn.org/cgi-bin/freida/freida.cgi

Journal of the American Medical Association
Like Academic Medicine, *JAMA* frequently contains articles regarding graduate medical education, including an annual report issue.

Each of these publications may be obtained from the AMA by writing to the following address:

American Medical Association
ATTN: Order Department
515 North State Street
Chicago, IL 60610
(312) 464-5000
http://www.ama-assn.org/

In addition, the following organizations may be contacted for further information:

American Board of Medical Specialties
1007 Church Street
Suite 404
Evanston, IL 60201-5913
Voice: (847) 491-9091
Fax: (847) 328-3596

Accreditation Council for Graduate Medical Education
515 North State Street
Chicago, IL 60611
(312) 464-4290

National Resident Matching Program
2501 M Street, NW
Suite 1
Washington, DC 20037-1307

Council of Medical Specialties Societies
51 Sherwood Terrace
Suite Y
Lake Bluff, IL 60044-2238
Phone: (847) 295-3456
Fax: (847) 295-3759

Educational Commission for Foreign Medical Graduates
3624 Market Street, 4th Floor
Philadelphia, PA 19104-2685
USA
Telephone: 215-386-5900

For further information on the American Osteopathic Association Intern Registration Program, contact National Matching Services Inc.:

National Matching Services Inc.
595 Bay St., Suite 301, Box 29
Toronto, Ontario
Canada, M5G 2C2
Telephone: (416) 977-3431
Fax: (416) 977-5020
or

National Matching Services Inc.
P.O. Box 1208
Lewiston, NY 14092-8208
Telephone: (716) 282-4013
Fax: (716) 282-0611

Medical Licensure

During your residency you will be required to become licensed to practice medicine in the state of your residency. No national agency grants unrestricted license to practice medicine throughout the United States. Instead, you must obtain a license from the medical board of the state where you are in training and where you plan to practice after completion of residency training (if they are different). Each state is independent in determining who may practice within the state and may have special requirements or restrictions for licensure.

Contact the Federation of State Medical Boards of the U.S., Inc. (FSMB) at the following address to obtain general information on medical licensure:

FSMB
400 Fuller Wiser Road, Suite 300
Euless, Texas 76039
(817) 868-4000
www.fsmb.org

Internet Resources

There are an increasing number of resources available on the Internet that can provide information about residencies, the matching process, and medical education in general. Access to these sites and the information contained in them are available without cost or special registration. Some areas of the ERAS and NRMP sites are restricted to participant and require a identification number and password (PIN). General information is available at these sites without special access privileges.

The American Association of Medical Colleges maintains an excellent Internet Web site with information about graduate medical education. Of particular interest may be the information it provides about the cost of undergraduate and graduate medical education. This information may be found at:

http://www.aamc.org/meded/edres/start.htm

The AMA also maintains the Fellowship and Residency Electronic Interactive Database (FREIDA) Web site at:

http://www.ama-assn.org/cgi-bin/freida/freida.cgi

An independent Web site that lists residencies is:

http://www.webcom.com/~wooming/residenc.html

If you are interested in the text of a *JAMA* article on the new match algorithm put in place in 1997, you can find it on the Web at:

http://www.pitt.edu/~alroth/jama2.html

The full citation for the test is: Roth AE, Peranson E, The effects of the change in the NRMP matching algorithm. JAMA 1997;278:729-732.

For a detailed accounting of how the match algorithm was constructed see:

http://www.pitt.edu/~alroth/phase1.html

Algorithms used to perform the matching of applicants to positions based on mutual preferences have been the subject of considerable research in the fields of mathematics and economics. An excellent source of technical information on this subject within the broader field of game theory, including an extensive bibliography on two-sided matching, can be obtained from:

http://www.economics.harvard.edu/~aroth/alroth.html

The Canadian Residency Matching Service maintains a comprehensive Web site that will be of interest to Canadian students and those considering postgraduate programs in Canada:

http://www.carms.ca/index.htm

The San Francisco Matching Program maintains a comprehensive Web site that will be of interest to students interested in careers in ophthalmology, otolaryngology, neurology, neurosurgery, and plastic surgery:

http://www.sfmatch.org/

The San Francisco Matching Program has information about the Central Application Service at this site:

http://www.sfmatch.org/general/CAS.html

For those interested in more information about the American Urological Association and its matching program information is available at:

http://www.auanet.org/

Or you may receive more information regarding the Urology Match from:
AUA Residency Matching Program
2425 West Loop South, Suite 333
Houston, Texas 77027-4207

The American Osteopathic Association Opportunities directory of internship and residency positions is available on the AOA's Web site:

www.aoa-net.org.

The Educational Commission for Foreign Medical Graduates (ECFMG) maintains a comprehensive Web site for graduates of medical schools outside the United States, Canada and Puerto Rico:

http://www.ecfmg.org/

References of Interest

Aranha GV. The international medical graduate in US academic general surgery. Arch Surg 1998;133:130-3.

Arnold RM, Landau C, Nissen JC, Wartman S, Michelson S. The role of partners in selecting a residency. Acad Med 1990;65:211-5.

Batchelor AJ. The residency interview. J Am Med Wom Assoc 1985;40:42, 61.

Berg D, Cerletty J, Byrd JC. The impact of educational loan burden on housestaff career decisions. J Gen Intern Med 1993;8:143-5.

Bickel J. Maternity leave policies for residents: an overview of issues and problems. Acad Med 1989;64:498.

Calkins EV, Willoughby TL, Arnold LM. Gender and psychosocial factors associated with specialty choice. J Am Med Wom Assoc 1987;42:170-2.

Colquitt WL. Medical specialty choice: a selected bibliography with abstracts. Acad Med 1993;68:391-436.

Crandall CS, Kelen GD. The influence of perceived risk of exposure to human immunodeficiency virus on medical student's planned specialty choices. Am J Emerg Med 1993;11:143-8.

DeForge BR, Richardson JP, Stewart DL. Attitudes of graduating senior at one medical school toward family practice. Fam Med 1993;25:111-3.

Dial TH, Elliot PR. Relationship of scholarships and indebtedness to medical students' career plans. J Med Educ 1987;62:316-24.

Dunn MR, Miller RS. The shifting sands of graduate medical education. JAMA 1996;276:710-3.

Fincher RM, Lewis LA, Rogers LQ. Classification model that predicts medical students' choices of primary care or non-primary care specialties. Acad Med 1992;67:324-7.

Fox M. Medical student indebtedness and choice of specialization. Inquiry 1993;30:84-94.

Gary NE, Soho MM, Shafron ML, Wald MK, Ben-David MF, Kelly WC. Graduates of foreign medical schools: progression to certification by the Educational Commission for Foreign Medical Graduates. Acad Med 1997;72:17-22.

Gayed NM. Residency directors' assessments of which selection criteria best predicted the performance of foreign-born foreign medical graduates during internal medicine residencies. Acad Med 1991;66:699-701.

Gong H Jr, Parker NH, Apgar FA, Shank C. Influence of the interview on ranking in the residency selection process. Med Educ 1984;18:366-9.

Grum CM, Wooliscroft JO. Choosing a specialty: a guide for students. JAMA 1993;269:1183, 1186.

Iserson KV. A medical career: idealism and reality. JAMA 1991;265:1190.

Kuhlmann TP, Fang WL, Fan Y. Physicians' view on how specialty-specific the first year of residency should be. Acad Med 1991;66:237-9.

McLaughlin MA, Daugherty SR, Rose WH, Goodman LJ. The impact of medical school debt on postgraduate career and lifestyle. Acad Med 1991;66:S43-5.

Metheny WP, Ling FW, Mitchum M. What to expect from a residency program? Answers from a directory of residency programs in obstetrics and gynecology. Obstet Gynecol 1998;91:311-4.

Part HM, Markert RJ. Predicting the first-year performances of international medical graduates in an internal medicine residency. Acad Med 1993;68:856-8.

Pecora AA. Factors influencing osteopathic physicians' decisions to enter in allopathic residency programs. J AM Osteopath Assoc 1990;90:527-33.

Potts MJ, Brazeau NK. The effects of first clinical clerkship on medical students' choices. Med Educ 1989;23:413-5.

Regan-Smith MG, Dietrich AJ, Olson AL, Moore-West M, Argenti PA. Teaching communication and interviewing skills to medical students preparing for residency interviews. J Med Ecuc 1988;63:801-3.

Richards P. Living Medicine: Planning a Career: Choosing a specialty. Cambridge: Cambridge University Press, 1990.

Rogers LQ, Fincher RM, Lewis LA. Factors influencing medical students to choose primary care of non-primary care specialties. Acad Med 1990;65(9 suppl):S47-8.

Sakala EP. Medical students' concerns about malpractice liability as a negative factor in specialty choice. Acad Med 1993;68:702-3.

Schwartz AL. Will competition change the physician workforce? Early signals from the market. Acad Med 1996;71:15-22.

Schwartz RW, Haley JV, Williams C, et al. The controllable lifestyle factor and students' attitudes about specialty selection. Acad Med 1990;65:207-10.

Simmonds AC, Robbins JM, Brinker MR, Rice JC, Kerstein MD. Factors important to students in selecting a residency program. Acad Med 1990;65:640-3.

Sklar DP, Tandberg D. The value of self-estimated scholastic standing in residency selection. J Emerg Med 1995;13:683-5.

Slick GL. Recruiting interns and residents to an osteopathic medical training program. J Am Osteopath Assoc 1992;92:654-56.

Stein J. Impact on personal life key to choosing a medical specialty in the '80's. Intern Med World Rep 1988;3:7.

Sutnick AI, Stilman PL, Norcini JJ, et al. Pilot study of the use of the ECFMG clinical competence assessment to provide profiles of clinical competencies of graduates of foreign medical schools for residency directors. Acad Med 1994;69:65-7.

Taylor CA, Weinstein L, Mayhew HE. The process of resident selection: a view from the
    residency director's desk. Obstet Gynecol 1995;85:299-303.

Valente J, Rappaport W, Neumayer L, Witzke D, Putnam CW. Influence of spousal
    opinions on residency selection. Am J Surg 1992;163:596-8.

Wagoner NE, Suriano R, Stoner JA. Factors used by program directors to select
    residents. J Med Educ 1986;61:10.

Walters BC. Why don't more women choose surgery as a career? Acad Med
    1993;68:350-1.

Xu G, Rattner SL, Veloski JJ, et al. The national study of the factors influencing men and
    women physicians' choices of primary care specialties. Acad Med 1995;70:398-404.

Zeldow PB, Daugherty SR. Personality profiles and specialty choices of students from
    two medical school classes. Acad Med 1991;66:283-7.

Zeldow PB, Devens M, Daugherty SR. Do person-oriented medical students choose
    person-oriented specialties? Do technology-oriented medical students choose
    technology-oriented specialties? Acad Med 1990;65(9 suppl):S45-6.

Zeldow PB, Preston RC, Daugherty SR. The decision to enter a medical specialty: timing
    and stability. Med Educ 1992;26:327-32.

Index